Healthy Foods

An irreverent
guide to
understanding
nutrition
and
feeding
your
family well

Healthy Foods

An irreverent
guide to
understanding
nutrition
and
feeding
your
family well

Leanne Ely C.N.C.

CHAMPION PRESS, LTD

CHAMPION PRESS, LTD.
FOX POINT, WISCONSIN

ISBN 1-891400-20-7

Manufactured in the United States of America 10 9 8 7 6 5

Book Design by Kathy Campbell, Wildwood Studios

Dedication

This book is dedicated to my own family—Scott, Caroline and Peter

Acknowledgments

Many thanks to some very special people who made this book possible—

The first acknowledgement has to go to my mentor, Cheri Swanson, C.N.C. for planting the seed, watering the plant and encouraging it to grow. You are a fountain of wisdom, Cheri.

To Debi Hough—thanks for believing in this book before even seeing it. Gosh, thanks for believing in me! We've had many a CR moment, hmm? If it wasn't for you....Q

And to Brook Noel—my favorite manic editor who deserves the Congressional Medal of Honor for putting up with computer ineptitude, endless email and manic questions.

To the taste testers, all thirty of you—thank you for your amazing patience. You made these recipes better than ever and I thank you for your help, cooking and tasting. You are all so special!

Contents

Why Another Healthy Cookbook?

Ten years ago, when my daughter Caroline was about nine months old (and I was breastfeeding less and feeding food more) she began to get ear infections. Like a good mother, I bundled her up and trundled off to the pediatrician's office. One magical prescription later, she was well. At least for a while. About two months later, she got sick again. Once again we visited the pediatrician's office, and left with another prescription for antibiotics. This cycle kept up for about four visits till I noticed a distinct pattern emerging and the doctor started hinting about tubes and prophylactic doses of antibiotics. At this point, my baby had dark circles under her eyes, a constant runny nose and an annoying little cough—none of which the pediatrician addressed.

I knew nothing except that round after round of antibiotics wasn't helping. I reached my limit after one particular visit. I was waiting for the elevator with my sick child, my purse on my shoulder, the prescription in my hand. I was distraught. I knew somehow that continuing antibiotics wasn't going to make this go away. As the elevator door opened, I crumbled the prescription up in my hand and threw it away in the trash can next to the elevator. I had no idea what I was going to do next, but I wasn't going to do something that clearly wasn't working.

Thus began my journey into wellness. I read everything I could get my hands on and became in my own pediatrician's vernacular, "a quack". But my quackery was working and my daughter was well. Two years and another baby later, I obtained my certification after Cheri Swanson, a nutritionist and friend, guided me through the process. I began helping other moms discover the importance of taking a personal, vested interest in their child's health and exploring other options besides medications, surgeries or breathing treatments. I had the pleasure of seeing one mom cancel a sinus surgery her daughter was scheduled for, watched a few other children go off breathing treatments and declared asthma free by their physicians, and saw countless potential tube surgeries canceled. All of these children had the same thing in common as my daughter. They were allergic to milk and the doctors never saw it. Once off milk, these kids' symptoms went away, their appearances improved and their dispositions were cheerful and sunny again.

But it wasn't just the kids I saw who were getting well and doing better. Everyone in the family was enjoying a much better level of health and benefiting from these important and healthy changes. Our family was no different. Everyone but my daughter still ate dairy products with no ill affect, but we certainly cleaned up our act as far as trying to eat organically and increasing the number of fresh foods we ate. I also noticed that our tastes began to change. The once craved ice cream, donuts and candies packed with coloring and other unmentionables weren't so attractive anymore. Sure we still had our treats—but we learned moderation.

I also noticed that I lost a few pounds of baby fat (I had just had my second child) and it wasn't as tough to lose as it was with my first. All in all, we felt great. These little changes, and this new awareness made its mark on our lives and on our health. There was no need to sell this family on whole foods and conscientious eating. We were there.

This is a book for parents about being in control of their child's health through responsible nutrition. What you don't know can hurt you and your child. Becoming a proactive parent and making that first scary step was the best thing I ever did for my family's health. And today, all these years later, if you're willing, I'll go with you as you take your first step.

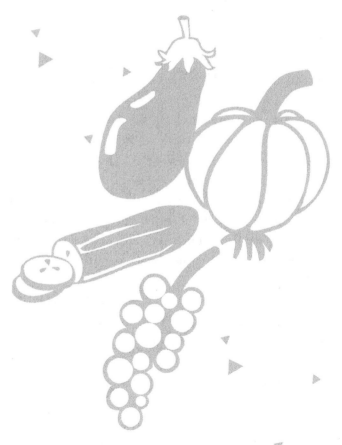

PART ONE

Realistic Health for Realistic Families

CHAPTER ONE

Change Your Food, Change Your Life

When people make changes in their lives, it is for compelling reasons. You move to another state. Why? Your spouse was transferred. That is a compelling reason. You change hairdressers. Why? The last one permed your hair into an Annie-do and gave you blisters on your scalp. That's compelling, too.

But it's not like that with food. Usually. Nothing stands out. Sure, you're tired and run down by 2:00 every day. Compelling? Not quite. You've tried a number of different "diets" only to never really get to the "Promised Land" the guru was telling you about. That's certainly not even close to compelling. What makes *Healthy Foods* different?

The biggest difference in what I am proposing is what you will add to the quality of your life and your family's life. In essence, I am handing you a value proposition here—the two biggest values in life are your health and your time and this book has the ability to impact both areas significantly.

I have noticed for myself that making changes doesn't work if someone is asking me to spend huge amounts of time and effort to make it happen. I won't ask that of you. Weigh and measure for a moment what you know to be true. Sugar burns you out—that is not great, big new news. But did you know that carbohy-drates, even the good, complex carbohydrates that you've been told are so good for you, are going to do the same if you consume too many? Too much protein holds the key to ill health, too, with kidney stones and renal failure both being associated with excessive protein intake. You can't eat just chicken, meat or even legumes and grains if you're a vegetarian, and expect to have robust health. It just doesn't work that way.

I don't know one person who doesn't want to reduce the time they spend on non-essential things. Time is the most valuable commodity we have. Health is right in there, too. Together, these two assets make the top one percent of everyone's list of things they wish they had more of. Everyone wants more time. Everyone wants better health. I say both are doable. Very doable, as a matter of fact.

I will mention over and over again in the next few chapters, how important it is to constantly be balancing what you eat. The balance being carbohydrates and protein and eating good sources of these foods; not crummy, junky ones. The key word here is balance. Your car needs gas and oil—not one or the other or one over the other. Both in equal balance, whatever that balance is for that particular car to run.

I have a $200 juicer in my cupboard. Why did I get

it? Because I wanted the excellent health benefits that juicing offered. Does it save me time? No. If you'll notice, I said it is in my cupboard and not sitting on my counter. I am sure there are plenty of people who spend their time juicing and for them, it's a good investment of time. At my house, the jury is still out and the juicer still sits in a dark cupboard. I am no different than anyone else—I need to have a payoff on both my time and my bottom line—the bottom line this time being health.

I feel without a shadow of a doubt, that learning balance was the best thing I ever did nutritionally speaking. As a nutritionist, my teaching was more along the lines of a high carbohydrate, low protein tack. One of the books I had to read was essentially a very low-fat, low protein, vegan-type diet. I read every "compelling" fact this guy dished out and came up empty handed. Why? Because 1) I knew my own body and I needed more than this guy was offering. 2) I didn't have that kind of time or money to juice, chop, cut, hunt and cook my food. 3) I wanted meatloaf and chicken pot pie for dinner and so did my family.

Change doesn't have to be weird, inconvenient or hard to do. For me, saving time and giving my family the best shot at a healthy lifestyle is of premium importance. And that is exactly what this book is all about.

Besides, I have a killer chicken pot pie recipe you've just gotta try.

CHAPTER TWO

A Health Plan for Real Life

Wouldn't it be great to have an easy formula for calculating exactly what your body needs? The FDA believes they have done just that. Just follow the food pyramid—one size fits all. If you did that, you would be eating six to 11 slices of bread a day. Not red hot if you have a carbohydrate sensitivity.

Then there are the "experts". The problem with "expert" opinions is that they vary like the wind. Protein is good, says one. Protein is bad, says another. Too much, too little, eat more, eat less, cook it, don't cook it, juice it, wear it. Forget it.

I believe that the person inhabiting the body is the best judge of what the body needs and how much. Obviously, if you are a woman that is 5'2" tall and you weigh 200 pounds, your judgment might be questionable. But with a realistic assessment of your own situation, a desire to live by what's best for you and not the latest guru, I believe it is possible to regain lost ground.

There is a starting place for everyone. A place to begin that will get you where you need to go— whether it's losing weight, maintaining your weight or just plain feeling better. It's time to get down to brass tacks and get to know your body all over again. Think for a minute. Do you feel better after a whole grain breakfast or an egg breakfast? Would you prefer to eat later? Earlier? A lot at one sitting or a little bit here and there throughout the day? The whole idea behind actually trusting your own body and not some expert is foreign to many people. But here we sit under this teaching, latest book or whatever, and swallow it whole—hook, line and sinker. We are reading away about eating only fresh fruit in the morning and agreeing to do this, knowing full well, we'll be ready to pass out before noon. We read about "combining" foods and forever giving up a favorite sandwich because the "combination" is wrong. Complete and utter hogwash! Who's the expert here? YOU are! We all know what we tolerate best, we know what we don't do well with. However, like lemmings at the end of a cliff willing to jump to their death, we ignore ourselves and look to the experts. It is only now in this day and age with all these so-called experts everywhere, that we as a society have had such a horrendous problem with eating disorders—whether they be overeating, under eating or throwing up what you're eating. I think we have spent far too much time, energy, money and navel gazing trying to figure this all out. We simply need to scrap it all and start over.

What does starting over look like, anyway? In a nutshell, it's following the food guide given at the end of this chapter. All the stuff listed is good for you. The amount you eat is going to be up to you. I'll give you a couple of guidelines and you can take it from there. I must tell you, my temptation is to tell you to eat this much protein, that much carbohydrates and this much fat. However, I am a victim myself of eight million experts telling me how to "do it"—whether it be high protein, low carbohydrates, low carbs, high protein, food combining, vegetarian, you name it—been there, done that. I have gained, lost, gained, lost, and done it all over again. I have listened to everyone else except the keeper of the body—me. Shouldn't I know what makes me feel better? Shouldn't I be in touch enough to know what works and what doesn't? You bet! We all need to have a basic understanding of nutrition, and we all need to know what constitutes healthy and what doesn't. But that's enough information, already. Doing healthy things, changing and moderating your own energy levels and well-being is the best way to stay on an even keel and keep some change in your pocketbook. You won't be running out to every guru that passes by with the latest and greatest "breakthrough". Instead, you will have taken the time to figure out what works best for you and your family by finding the "guru" within.

Hippocrates, the father of medicine, said, "Let food be your medicine. Medicine your food." How much better off we would all be had we heeded those words of wisdom so many years ago. What we eat directly affects the quality of health we enjoy (or don't enjoy) today. Quality nutrition is the barest basic of good health. There isn't a soul on earth who doesn't need the basic nutrients: protein, carbohydrates, fats and water. By choosing excellent sources for these basics, your body is able to perform and function at its best. Let's examine the cornerstones of solid nutrition.

Protein

Protein is the quality building material needed to produce cells in the body. It is absolutely essential for everyone to include protein in their diet. There has been a lot of debate in recent years on the amount of protein necessary, and the debate will probably continue. The place we always come back to is balance. You need protein, but it must be balanced with the other nutrients, too.

Amino acids, the product of protein being broken down in the body, are what fuel body function. The body is constantly in process, and amino acids are key to its function. There is much more to this amino acid thing, like essential and non-essential amino acids and what that all means, but the important thing to know about amino acids is that they come from protein: meat, chicken, fish, dairy products, eggs. Also beans, rice, grains and nuts provide protein, although not complete like meat, chicken, etc. To make a complete protein, you need to combine the bean with a grain, nut or rice.

Carbohydrates

If proteins are like bricks for a house, carbohydrates are like gas to a car. This is the stuff that makes us go!

The best quality carbs are found in vegetables, beans and grains—these would be considered complex carbohydrates. They are more complicated molecularly speaking, and take longer for the body to process. Kind of like putting a green log on a hot fire—it'll burn, but it may take a while. Simple carbs are also called simple sugars: fruit is a simple sugar, for example. Simple sugars are like throwing a dry, well-cured piece of wood on the flame. It burns hotly, quickly and supplies a fast boost of energy to the fire.

Carbohydrates are converted into glucose for either immediate use or for later. If it is to be used later, it gets stored in the liver, becoming glycogen. This is important to know because we are a culture of carbo loving addicts, who continually bombard our poor livers with an overload of glycogen. If the glycogen stores become too much, they convert to fat. Not pretty. Just remember that next time you're tempted to binge on carbs. Your storehouse may be full and you could be sitting on those extra carbs tomorrow.

Another part of the carbohydrate family is fiber. Fiber is non-nutritive, but provides essential function to the body: cleaning. Roto-rooter action. Fiber can be had in several different forms: pectin, lignin, bran, hemicellulose, cellulose and mucilages. Gross sounding names, all with different functions. For example, bran does the clean sweep number on your digestive tract, while pectin acts like a sponge. Mucilages help to keep blood sugar levels regulated. Hemicellulose and cellulose also aid in absorption. Lignin is beneficial in lowering cholesterol. Eating foods with different fiber sources is really optimal for health. And it's easy to do, if you choose to eat a good variety of vegetables, fruit and grains. There's no need in worrying which type of fiber fits where, or what food has what, if fruit, vegetables and grains are a big part of your diet.

The typical American diet is so sadly lacking in anything remotely resembling fiber. White bread, white rice, white, white, white. This stuff has all had the fiber pulled out and isn't worth a nickel nutritionally. Putting fiber back in your diet will make a huge difference in your health. And your colon will really appreciate it, too.

Fats

Fat isn't bad. Fat is good. It's only bad to eat too much of the wrong kind. It is a necessary component to normal brain development in children. It is an energy powerhouse and helps the body with the work of growth. However, after about two years of age, our fat requirement is dramatically reduced.

I don't think it necessary to expound on the problem of too much fat in the diet. It sort of makes its presence known in our lives, if you catch my drift. The question is: what kind of fat do we need and how much?

To understand fats better, let's take a quick look at the types of fats: saturated, polyunsaturated, and mono-unsaturated. Saturated fats are found in anything from an animal—poultry, meat or dairy. The only exception would be palm oil, coconut oil and hydrogenated anything—like Crisco. Polyunsaturated fats are found in plants like corn, soybean and safflower oils. We've all seen the commercials on vegetable oils helping HDL ("good" cholesterol) levels. Monounsaturated oils are found primarily in nuts and plants, too. Olive oil is a good example of an excellent monounsaturated oil.

Trans-fatty acids are also getting a lot of press right now. They are the black sheep of the fat family. Good examples are margarines and shortenings. Ditch this stuff and get yourself some real butter and good oil. Yes, I am giving you permission to eat butter. It may be a saturated fat, but at least it's real food and not some plasticized pretend stuff, with fake-o coloring, artificial flavoring and a lousy taste.

Water: The Beverage of Choice

Fact is, we don't drink enough water. But we're a thirsty bunch—just look at the soft drink size you can get at your nearest convenience store. A "Super Gulp" or whatever they're called in your neck of the woods, holds 32 ounces of soft drink. Just think, you can drink a whole quart of cola and still be thirsty!

And you will be thirsty, too. The only thing that will truly quench that thirst is water. Water makes up 70% of the human body. Almost every body function uses water. Water carries the good stuff in, water takes the bad stuff out. Water maintains body temperature and helps the circulatory system. Water is absolutely essential and yet, most everyone's body is screaming for it. Still, we turn a deaf ear and order another Super Gulp.

So, how do we go from a partially dehydrated state to one of hydration when we didn't even know we were dehydrated in the first place? Water drinking is a good habit that needs to be developed. It's kind of like wearing a seat belt—until you are in the habit of doing so, it feels awkward. But after that habit is developed, you'd feel funny driving without your seat belt on. And so it is with the habit of water drinking. Drinking water at the end of the day is asking for trouble—and a poor night's sleep from all the bathroom trips. Try drinking it instead of the usual soft drinks, teas and coffees. Try drinking it as you go along in the day—one glass before a meal and one glass after a meal will give you six glasses of water. Stick another on each end of your day, right when rising and an hour before bed and you've made "quota". Yes, the old standard 8 8-ounce glasses of water a day is a good guideline. You can also self-check to make sure you're doing okay by this simple potty test: your urine should be light colored and not dark yellow. That is a good barometer of how much water you need. If you're a marathon runner, for example, you will need more. On the other hand, if you are older and not very active and petite, maybe six glasses is plenty.

But don't just turn on the tap and start filling your glass. Tap water has turned into a game of Russian roulette: who knows what you'll get in your tap water? All kinds of contaminants, from chemicals to heavy metals, to added chlorine and fluoride, present problems.

While chlorine may help get your whites their whitest white, it isn't something you want to drink. Chlorine does kill bacteria, no doubt about that. If you were stranded in the mountains with your jug of Clorox, you could rest assured that the water you treated with chlorine would be safer to drink than stream water.

However, voluntarily drinking chlorinated water is something you may wish to avoid. High levels of chlorine byproducts are known carcinogens, and unfortunately, the level of chlorine in drinking water today can be quite high, creating an atmosphere for these byproducts to proliferate.

Fluoridation is something that everyone thinks is pretty nifty. I beg to differ. True, dentists treat kids' teeth with fluoride to prevent cavities, toothpastes have it and yes, it's in the drinking water, too. Although it is a naturally occurring substance, there are problems associated with added fluoride. Excessive use of fluoride creates fluorine, a poisonous by-product of fluoride, to build up in the body. Fluorine can have detrimental effects on the immune system. Not only that, but the *Clinical Toxicology of Commercial Products* shows that fluoride is more poisonous than lead, although slightly less poisonous than arsenic. It is not a comforting thought to know that your child's toothpaste is just slightly less poisonous than arsenic.

Chronic use of fluoride can also result in osteoporosis.

The Journal of the American Medical Association published three separate articles from 1990 to 1992 that indicted fluoride in the water for the increase in hip fractures. In the respected *New England Journal of Medicine,* the March 22, 1990 issue linked fluoride treatment of osteoporosis to increased hip fractures and bone fragility. Over fluoridation can discolor and blotch children's teeth—my own daughter's mottled teeth tell that story.

Bottled water may seem like a good idea and for the most part, it is better than tap water. However, with most states not having a true regulating system in place, there is no telling what you may be getting. For all intents and purposes, bottled water "from the mountains" could be tap water from a city located in the mountains. And that "natural spring" water that you bought, could come from anywhere, since there is no legal definition of the word "spring".

Filtered water is another avenue when looking for pure water. Filtration devices abound from multi-level marketing companies to hardware stores and discount stores. Many claims are made with these devices and it's hard to know what to choose. The guideline for buying a water filter depends on what you are trying to accomplish. For removal of chlorine and fluoride, a simple water treatment jug you can buy at your discount store will suffice. Check the box before purchasing it to see what it can and cannot do. There are, of course, many different ways to get your water just right. How you go about it will depend on your financial resources and what's important to your family's health goals. We use a Brita-type water system and though I know I could have a bigger, better and more expensive system, this is adequate for us.

The Guidelines

Remember everyone's needs are different! If this wasn't so, Eskimos, who traditionally eat about 11 pounds of fatty meat a day, would be lining the waiting rooms of cardiologists all over Alaska. But guess what? They aren't. They know what's best for them—they have the example of their heritage. Knowing your ancestory is one thing, but for most people a great deal of experimentation needs to take place.

Here is your Golden-Rule Guideline: Eat whole unprocessed foods and a balance of protein and complex carbs. Everyone knows the Golden Rule—to do unto others as you would have others do unto you. Taking this principle and applying it to nutrition makes perfect sense: your body will definitely "do unto you" if you don't take care of it. On the other hand, it will take care of you, if you take care of it. It's simple and relatively painless. By following this guideline you will be one step closer to getting a perfect fit nutritionally. Losing weight, gaining weight, your moods, feeling "satisfied and full"—all of these things need to come into play as you go along. You needn't worry about doing this with a whole household either. I can't imagine trying to cook all day like a short order cook according to everyone's needs! Just watch, look and listen. I have one child that would eat nothing but complex carbs if I let her, but she falls apart if she doesn't have adequate protein in her diet. I am usually trying to insure that there is some almond butter on her

whole wheat bread or that she's eaten a good-sized piece of cheese with her bread. My son, on the other hand, has a better gauge on what makes him feel good and he will often seek out a protein-rich snack or ask for an extra portion of protein after a particularly strenuous day of exercise (like after baseball practice). Not all families need to be as on top of it as we are to insure this amount of protein is present. This is a critical element in my own family's balancing act. As you explore the Golden Rule as it applies to your family—you'll discover how to best customize your balancing act to meet your family's needs.

Most of us have distorted our taste buds, stretched out our stomachs and indulged our appetites by having an anything-goes mentality. We like what we are eating, so we eat more. For fun, let's pretend we have just eaten a good-for-you meal. And like most people, we totally ignore the fact that we have had enough. The first clue was the portion—it was adequate and balanced: protein and complex carbohydrates. We aren't hungry anymore but we liked it, so what do we do? We have a second helping. On top of this, we are thirsty and we don't even know it. We ignore our body's many cries for water and walk around dehydrated. Even though the stomach isn't giving the groaning from Thanksgiving signal, if we gave ourselves a few minutes and had a glass of water, we'd know we are adequately full!

So here they are, the guidelines for healthy eating. A bounty of wonderful things; some of which are probably your favorites:

The Golden Rule

Eat whole unprocessed foods and a balance of protein and complex carbs.

Choose your balance of foods from the categories below.

PROTEIN SOURCES:

Eggs, meat and poultry, salmon and tuna, (other fish are fine, too)
dairy products, soy products, legumes
(try to eat free-range eggs and poultry, and organically raised meats)

CARBOHYDRATES:

Whole grains, brown rice, vegetables and fruits

FATS:

Cold-pressed mono-unsaturated oils, like safflower oil, properly stored,
as well as olive oil and flax oil.
Butter, unsalted and organic if possible, used very sparingly.

BEVERAGES:

Pure, preferably filtered water. Freshly squeezed juice, but not more than a glass a day.

Coffee or tea in very limited amounts—a cup or two a day.

CHAPTER THREE

Qualifying Your Food

Quality nutrition can only come from quality food. Quality food is defined as less processed, more natural, more basic foods—like fresh fruits, vegetables, whole grains, etc. Easy stuff to get at the market.

There are however, concerns that we are necessarily, having to deal with in this 21st century. The problems of pesticide residues, genetically engineered food, irradiation and hormone-fed, antibiotic-inoculated chicken and beef, plague consumers today. And most consumers don't even know there is anything to be concerned about going on with their food. All of these alterations to our food, which are supposedly "safe" for parents and their growing children, have been blessed by governmental agencies and special interest groups.

The point here isn't to start something, but to give enough information to families that they may make their own decisions on how to proceed on their individual pathways to health. While this controversial information is available to the public, you have to do some digging to find it. This is not the stuff one finds on the front page of daily newspapers.

Let's start with pesticides. Pesticide use has been out of control for many years. In her whistle-blowing book *Silent Spring*, Rachel Carson showed the world exactly what irresponsible use of pesticides did to the environment. Before

this book, the public never really questioned the validity or safety of pesticide use. Though Rachel's book was ground-breaking in many ways, what is going on today would have Rachel turning in her grave.

Because of Rachel's efforts, an awareness was formed that helped get dichlorodiphenyltrichloro-ethane, better known as DDT, banned from the U.S. in the early 70's. Though banned in the U.S., DDT is still being produced and sold to Third World countries. They use this deadly substance in their agriculture, as well as to control the spread of malaria. This is happening right now today, almost 30 years after this carcinogen was taken off the shelves. Even worse, private companies in the United States produce this killer and sell it to these countries. That's like giving a child a loaded weapon to play with.

But there is more to this problem than just pesticides. Agriculture today spends millions on artificial fertilizers, fungicides, herbicides and rodentcides, as well as pesticides. The average tomato has been picked too young, bombarded with as many as 15 different pesticides and fungicides, pummeled with ripening agents and artificially colored and waxed to appeal to the eye. It's been grown in artificially fertilized soil and could actually have some salmon genes included in this motley chemical mix! We'll get to the salmon genes in a minute...

Before we go any further, we need to know how this affects health or does it? And what about the farmer's bottom line? Is this the only option for him?

According to a June, 1998, article in *Acres USA,* organic farmers have shown a higher nutrient content to their produce about 40% of the time, comparing to conventional crops only showing a higher content about 15% of the time. This is based on more than 30 studies comparing nutrient content of organic and non-organic produce, with a comparison of over 300 individual nutrients.

The dangers of pesticides? I believe there is substantial evidence to show the wisdom of eating as organically as possible. Of course pesticides are dangerous—just ask the bugs. Do they wash off? If they did, don't you think it's kind of silly for the farmer to apply them in the first place? Every time they irrigated, they would be literally washing their money down the drain.

The crop yields to the farmer could be the same, a little less or in some cases, more. According to a May/June 1997 article in *Organic Gardening,* a study conducted by Ohio State University discovered that the European corn borer moth lays 18 times more eggs on sweet corn plants grown in chemical soils than in organic soils. Though one study isn't completely conclusive, it is quite interesting. Environmentally speaking, there is no question as to which is the superior method. Organically raised produce is much more earth-friendly. Organic farmers are making money, just as their traditional counterparts, it's just a different way of doing business.

Genetically engineered foods are another potential problem. Genetic engineering involves taking genes from one species and implanting it to another. This becomes a sort of Frankenstein-like creation, making an ordinary tomato the recipient of salmon traits, for example. It might seem like a neat idea, implanting extra nutrition into your average tomato, but it's more complicated than that.

We need to understand genetics a little bit. Genes don't necessarily control a single trait. It is possible that a gene can control several different traits in a plant. It would be easy to allow an undesirable trait to slip through the cracks of the global ecosystem creating who-knows-what. It's not like you can go back and clean up a little mess either—from that point on, it's here to stay. Scary thought.

The other problem with genetic engineering is instability. A humid environment in Florida may make the genetically altered tomatoes different then the tomatoes from cool, rainy Oregon. Who knows what you'll be getting in Albuquerque?

The FDA, USDA and EPA—all three of these powerhouse governmental agencies—regulate genetically engineered food. None of the agencies require any kind of public record on what farms are using genetically engineered seed. Distributors of produce who sell to food manufacturers and grocery stores, can mix regular crops with genetically engineered crops, so there's no way of knowing what you have. The problem becomes insurmountable should ever a health risk be discovered since there is no way to trace and fix it.

Food irradiation presents another set of problems. The idea behind food irradiation is to nuke the bacteria on different food to get rid of food-borne diseases. When you consider that well over six million people a year become ill from different types of food poisoning, etc., it seems logical. But the issue is: is it safe to radiate food?

Again, like the problem with genetic engineering, food irradiation presents the possibility for new substances to be created, causing who knows what kind of potential health problems. The vitamin content in food is changed: up to 10% of vitamins A, B1, E and K can be obliterated through irradiation. What's worse, is there have been no long-term human safety studies, although irradiation has been around for 40 years.

Another disturbing trend to be reckoned with is hormone treated livestock. While Americans and Canadians make a hefty profit off of estradiol-treated cattle, (a tidy $80/head more) the European Union has banned the importation of North American cattle that have been treated with this known cancer-causing estrogen.

The disturbing question is, why haven't we stopped North American cattle producers from using a known carcinogenic in their cattle producing? Because it's not a problem. At least according to the USDA and FDA, it's not.

But not everyone agrees. Estrogen-type hormones have been linked to all kinds of problems: from the early onset of puberty to different cancers of the reproductive system. The implications are huge, but so far, no one is stepping up to the line.

Steps to Change

I almost felt guilty including the information in this chapter. My passion for nutrition is to see people empowered to change and to become healthier by eating well. I recognize that information like this might paint a bleak picture. It is bleak if you do nothing with the information you now have. Remember though, that knowledge is power and there are always options.

Here are some important things you can do:

1 Buy organic. Yes, it's more expensive. But by buying organic, you are supporting organic farmers who are now kindred spirits: this little organic farmer is the guy who is going to effect the most change. Period. Have you noticed how it is getting easier and easier to find organic produce even in chain grocery stores? Buy organic as much as you are able. If you don't see organic in your local store, ask the manager to start carrying it.

2 Buy locally grown stuff from produce stands. Sure, it won't be organic, but you can bet it's been minimally bombarded by pesticides, won't be genetically engineered or irradiated and the prices are usually less than the grocery store. I would definitely stay away from produce grown in Mexico and South America.

3 Eat in season. Asparagus in December may seem gourmet, but where was it grown? Unless its hothouse varieties, chances are good this stuff was grown in places with less control over pesticides than the U.S. If you are not sure what is in season and what isn't, look at the prices. Grapes, melon and summer squash will be a lot less expensive during the summer than in the middle of January.

4 Grow some of your own. Seriously. It's not that hard. I had a teeny, tiny little strip of land around our home when we lived in Southern California that was full of impatiens, nasturium—lots of pretty flowers. In between these pretty flowers, I planted zucchini, green bush beans, summer squash and lettuces. We grew tomatoes in big pots on the front patio and prolific basil, too. So I didn't have a cornfield, big deal. I had an unbelievable bounty considering I had "nowhere" to put a garden.

5 See if there are **community gardens** in your town or vicinity. This is an inexpensive option for someone longing to stick their hands in the soil but are apartment-bound. There are often waiting lists, so sign up early.

Something else I have noticed, much to my delight, is the availability of antibiotic-free, hormone-free meats and poultry. Again, if you don't see it in your market, ask for it. Tell your friends to ask and effect change within your own community! They would rather carry it for you than lose you to the competition. Organic milk, butter and eggs are also available. Even with the higher prices, if you are shopping the way you should be and spending your money on quality rather than bulk, non-nutritional food, your food budget will probably stay the same. Mine actually came down! It's a matter of priorities—we always do what is important to us. The ability to effect change needn't be a political process.

Just remember, the squeaky wheel gets the grease. You should see what my market is carrying now...

Nutrient-packed Foods

Some food is simply better than other food. For example, filet of sole is good fish to eat, but salmon offers more nutrition. Salmon would be considered a nutrient-packed food. Not that you shouldn't eat filet of sole, it's just having the awareness that salmon is a better nutritional choice might have you choosing salmon over the sole next week at the market. Make sense? If, on the other hand, you despise salmon and even the pinkish color of salmon, by all means, get the sole!

When choosing nutrient-rich vegetables, look for the color. The dark green leafy types are almost always going to be more nutrient-packed than the whitish, pale green ones. The best thing I could say about Iceberg lettuce is that it is rich in water. Nutritionally, there is almost nothing there—especially compared to romaine, Boston, red leaf, salad bowl and spinach. You can build a gorgeous, nutritional salad using rich color as your guide: spinach, carrot, red onion, cucumber, tomato—do you see the difference? Compare that to a wedge of iceberg with a blob of bleu cheese dressing. Which one do you think is going to feed your body?

Use the Golden Rule Guidelines on page 21 as the basis for building your family's meals.

■■■

CHAPTER FOUR

Breaking It Down: making sense out of nutrition

Now that we understand the "whys" behind the importance of eating nutritiously and eating clean, quality food, let's break it down and assimilate how it effects your nutrition plan. First up, the famous protein vs. carbohydrate debate.

It is almost laughable how diets go in and out of vogue. Low-carb, high-protein may be hot this year, but next year it will be decried as passé and the "right" diet will be (again) high-carb, low-protein.

What utter nonsense. The fact is, we need both carbohydrate and protein. Not gobs of protein and no carbs or visa versa. As with most things in life, balance is key.

When you eat a balance of protein and carbohydrates, your body is on an even keel. The carbs provide the quick-to-assimilate fuel, while the protein will help sustain it. That is great news for those who suffer from hypoglycemic-type symptoms (low blood sugar). Protein evens out the carb thrust, if you will. Just to clarify, when we talk about carbohydrates here, we are talking about complex carbohydrates, not simple carbohydrates. With the exception of fruit, which is a simple carbohydrate, you should avoid simple carbohydrates. You do your body no favors when you send your blood sugar through the ceiling and your insulin levels surging. To abuse your body in this fashion habitually, will

put you one step closer to Type II Diabetes later in life, or in some cases, earlier. I cannot emphasize that enough. Simple carbohydrates, except for fruit, (but don't overdo it on the fruit, either) wreaks absolute havoc on your body and that of your child's, too. (If you don't know what a simple carbohydrate is, think white sugar. Better yet, think donut and degenerate your list from there.)

By keeping in mind that your goal for each meal is quality protein and quality complex carbohydrates, it is fairly simple to balance your diet. For breakfast, try a breakfast burrito—a whole wheat tortilla (complex carbohydrate) wrapped around some scrambled eggs (protein). For lunch, try a tuna (protein) pita pocket (complex carbs). At dinner, make it a point to balance out again—chicken, brown rice and some veggies. But remember that your balance will be unique to you. You may require more carbs or more protein. Your body will tell you if you listen.

Another area of continuing debate is over fat. Low fat, no fat, high fat even. Who can figure it all out? The "expert" opinions run the gamut and only make a confusing issue even more so. The fact is, we need a certain amount of fat to keep the machine (body) lubed up and operational. A little olive oil or other high quality oil in salad dressing for example, shouldn't be avoided. Eat-

FIVE GUIDELINES FOR YOUR JOURNEY

A couple of other guidelines that I think are important as you start this journey:

1. Be adventurous and daring! If you make this fun, your kids will, too.

2. Avoid making the sounds, "ewww"and "blech".

3. In like manner, avoid the words, "yuck" and "gross".

4. Try to make sure to include at least one raw thing a day: a salad or some fruit perhaps.

5. Buy your produce in season. I mentioned this before, but it's worth mentioning again.

Avoid like the plague, any appliance that says, "Fry Baby", "Fry Daddy" or any other kin of the Fry family. This appliance can be the ruination to your health. Fried anything is gross. (I can say that because I wrote the rules) Key words are: steamed, broiled, baked, sauteed (with minimal oil) but ixnay on the frying.

ing fatty fish like salmon, is another example of high quality fat. These are rich fats that supply the body with the "lube" power it needs in the form of EFA's—essential fatty acids.

To understand the importance of EFA's, let's start with the two basic types: omega-3 and omega-6. Omega-3 is found primarily in raw nuts and seeds, and supplements you can buy from the health food store like borage oil, grapeseed oil and primrose oil. Omega-6 on the other hand, is found mostly in deep water fish, like salmon, mackerel, herring and sardines. It can also be found in flax seed—both the oil and seeds are a particularly wonderful addition to anyone's diet.

EFA's play a vital role in keeping hair shiny and skin smooth. All kinds of dermatitis would benefit from a diet rich with EFA's. Not only do EFA's make for a prettier face, they may help with the treatment and prevention of PMS symptoms, especially the use of primrose oil. In addition, EFA's aid in the prevention of arthritis, keeping blood pressure low, and help keep triglyceride levels at bay. They also help transmit nerve impulses in the brain and are absolutely critical to brain function. No wonder your mom called fish, "brain food"—there is some truth to that.

And while olive oil and sesame seed oil may be good choices, the way they are made and stored are of primary concern. When you are buying any oil, look for the words, "expeller pressed" or "cold pressed". Expeller, or cold pressed oils, are made by pressing the oil through an mechanical expeller. No heat or chemicals are used, keeping the fatty acids intact. Health food stores for sure carry such oils and the regular grocery store is getting better about carrying healthy oils, too. Regular grocery store vegetable oils are expelled using chemicals and high heat, destroying any nutrients or EFA's. This isn't just tough luck in the nutrition department, it turns a benign food into a nutritional terrorist. The good fat has become bad fat—trans fatty acids. Trans fatty acids aren't just in soldified, hydrogenated oils—they are in products like regular vegetable oil whose delicate fatty acids have been throttled to get them out of their source.

But even after you buy cold pressed oil (olive oil is mostly a cold-pressed oil—although they are starting to process olive oil as well now), if it isn't stored correctly, it will become rancid. Those fatty acids are delicate and storing them at room temperature (yes, even olive oil) is a mistake. Just because your oil doesn't smell rancid, doesn't mean it isn't. It's just not smelly—yet. Think about it: do you think your oil just stays perfectly fine for weeks and months at a time and then one day goes rancid—poof—just like that? Of course not. It's just like having a ripe peach in your fruit bowl, over time, that peach breaks down till it's swarming with fruit flies, mushy and beyond eating. But it still smells good, even though it is one step away from the compost pile. And I seriously doubt I could talk you into eating it. Oil is just like that—as delicate as a ripe peach. Refrigeration is a must to keep it from going bad.

To Supplement or Not Supplement— An Important Question

If you have heard it once, you have probably heard it a hundred times: if you eat right you don't need to supple-

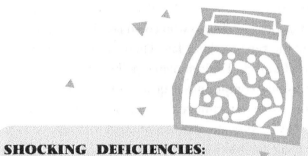

SHOCKING DEFICIENCIES:

1/3 of our children are deficient in iron

Over 90% are deficient in magnesium

One in six kids lack enough vitamin A

Almost ½ of children are seriously deficient in vitamin C

Almost ½ lack enough zinc

One in five children are deficient in folate

One in seven kids are deficient in vitamin B-12

Almost 1/3 of children are deficient in B-6

The *Vitamin Journal* came up with this shocking list. Just remember: you don't have car insurance because you plan on something happening. It's just the prudent thing to do to guarantee you're covered. And that's exactly what vitamins and supplements (when taken in the proper, directed dosages) are there for, too—simple coverage for when you don't get it right. And unless you're an exception, the rule is no one gets it right all the time.

ment with vitamins. Well, that's partly true. I have met precious few people who could lay claim to eating well all the time, without fail. There is more to just eating well though. Environmental pollutants, stress, and the possible compromised quality of food make supplements an unfortunate necessity in today's world.

A good quality, natural multiple vitamin is a logical choice for everyone, adults and children. Sort of an insurance policy against your lifestyle. Not in lieu of healthy eating, mind you, but as a supplementary source of vitamins and minerals. Ideally, a good mul-

Phytochemicals have been hailed by the press to be the latest and greatest nutritional discovery since vitamin C. And for good reason. Phytochemicals are the biologically active substances in plants that give them their color, disease resistance and flavor. There are many different phytochemicals in fruits and vegetables. For instance, in broccoli and other cruciferous vegetables, indoles are the phytochemical that is known to increase immune activity and help the body rid itself of toxins. Flavonoids, found in citrus and berries, form a barrier to prevent cancer-causing hormones from connecting to cells. A tomato may have as many as 10,000 different phytochemicals. Research has shown thus far, that the main purpose of phytochemcials is to fight cancer in one way or another. Obviously, a diet rich in phytochemically rich foods is a good move toward a much healthier lifestyle. We all know eating fruits and vegetables is good for you. Now you know why.

tiple should be rich in anti-oxidants as well as other vitamins and minerals. Try and avoid the mega-vitamins—most of that ends up in the toilet.

Taking a little extra vitamin C is also a good idea, considering the environmental pollutants that regularly bombard our every breath. Smokers especially, would be wise to increase their vitamin C. I am reluctant to recommend dosages, as I believe this is an area of controversy that is best avoided. I will go on record, however, and tell you that 60 mg. of vitamin C (minimum RDA) is too little. Linus Pauling, the Nobel Prize winner, regularly took about 10 grams of vitamin C a day. That may be a bit much, but he lived well into his 90's. In anything this important, it is always beneficial to seek qualified counsel and do your own research.

I hestitate to make hard and fast recommendations on vitamins, but I know a bad children's vitamin when I see one. Generally, if it's named after a cartoon and is full of artificial colorings and flavorings, it's something you definitely don't want. On the other hand, if it's a megawatt kid's vitamin from the health food store, it's also something you don't want. You need to look for a quality product (no artificial ingredients or fillers) with a gentler approach to nutrition, not supersonic dosage. I am partial to Shaklee's children's products because of those very reasons and their stuff is easily absorbed by young bodies. You need to remember that a supplement is just that—a supplement. The last thing you should try and do is supplant a crummy diet with a vitamin pill. It does not work, although it may assuage a guilty conscience momentarily.

PART TWO

Here's Looking at you, Kid

CHAPTER FIVE

Fat Kids, Fit Kids, Somewhere In-Between Kids

Six million kids are seriously overweight. So proclaims the cover of *Newsweek* magazine (July 3, 2000) with a picture of a kid going head-first into a drippy ice cream cone for all he's worth.

Six million kids seriously overweight is somewhat of a jaw-dropping statistic. The article later stated that there were five million kids behind these kids who were borderline obese.

Just a few decades ago, it was considered a sign of good health for kids to be a little bit chubby. But chubby has turned into tubby and these kids are at serious risk.

Heart problems, type II diabetes, asthma, elevated blood pressure, cholesterol problems—all stem from obesity. The fact is something can be done about this particular problem, but it's not easy. Even children who are genetically predisposed to obesity can still keep their weight under control. Consider children with a variety of illnesses, disabilities and impairments that require some sort of therapy to get better or overcome them. These kids work hard at their therapies with the hope that one day they will speak without a speech impediment or walk without crutches. The kids and families take this therapy seriously, investing both time and money in the process. They are committed to getting well or making improvements that will have a lasting affect on the child's health or well-being. If your child was in an accident, you would do what it takes to help him get well again. Is there any parent that wouldn't? Dealing with childhood obesity is not much different. It requires a commitment from the child and the parents to make this "therapy" work. The neat thing is, unlike other types of problems that require different therapies, this one's cure rate is 100 percent—if there is effort. The bad thing is if it's not "cured", in all likelihood, the child will develop into a fat adult with obesity as a lifelong issue.

Fast food is the bane of our society and has infiltrated our lifestyles. One pass through the drive-thru can give a kid his daily allotment in calories and double that of fat. Case in point: a super-sized meal at McDonald's packs over 1800 calories and a whopping 84 grams of fat. Fast food outlets have invaded big discount stores, gas stations and every corner—they're everywhere, including our schools. The worst part of this is that the educrats have caved to the almighty buck allowing these fast food, health-destroying icons into the schools! It's not the old cafeteria stand-by salisbury steak and gravy that's making your kids fat—it's the burgers, fried chicken and French fries that your child can get right

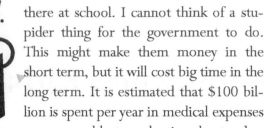

there at school. I cannot think of a stupider thing for the government to do. This might make them money in the short term, but it will cost big time in the long term. It is estimated that $100 billion is spent per year in medical expenses and lost production due to obesity related illness. Why, oh why can these people not connect the dots?

When I was in high school, we had a vending machine right next to the gym, that for a quarter, would give you a cold, red apple. I would love getting one of these after gym class. Nowadays, the vending machines are full of sodas, chips and candies. Unfortunately, most kids are overfed and undernourished. Gary Null, Ph.D., a noted nutritionist from New York calls this effect "negative nutrition"—a condition where the body is actually being robbed of nutrients while being fed. That's why these kids are so hungry—they haven't really had their bodies fed. The constant eating of junk is obvious evidence that their bodies are needy of some real food.

Not chips, not soda, cookies, or any of the other stuff consumed in mass quantity. Kids need good protein, a good, high quality complex carbohydrate and they need to drink water. Most likely, they are addicted to sugar and they need to be weaned off that, too. No diet necessary, no fat camp, no special exercises. Just good healthy food, moderate real kid exercise and the fat will fall off.

As a parent, our focus needs to be on feeding a soul, not filling a hole. Our children and ourselves, for that matter, are living, breathing souls that need real food to grow physically, spiritually, mentally and emotionally. Healthful growth occurs when the body is healthfully fed. Just like the old computer saying, garbage in, garbage out, it's not hard to figure out that feeding ourselves and our children poorly is going to produce sub-standard results.

I cannot think of one family that would knowingly pour less than quality fuel in their car's gas tank. Anything less would not only impair the car's performance, but could possibly damage the engine itself. Why would we knowingly give inferior fuel to our children?

Another important factor in conquering obesity is exercise. All too often, exercise has been replaced by sedentary activities like television watching, Nintendo and the computer. Physical Education and even recess are falling out of favor with schools in an attempt to become more competitive globally on the educational front. It's not uncommon for a child to spend 15 hours or more a week in front of the television. Thanks to the remote, they don't even have to get up to change the channel.

We are a non-TV watching family. That might seem

weird to a lot of people, but for us the TV was too much competition for our real priorities. It was just too easy to get sucked into its powerful, hypnotic glow, so we dumped it over three years ago. We still have it, but use it only as a video monitor, but even so, video watching is a special occasion. The computer is another place where we draw the line and we don't own any computer games, Nintendo or anything else like that. The kids do have a Geosafari though, a sort of computer-like contraption that allows them to learn all kinds of things. It's much like a computer game without the addiction factor. Pretty pedestrian equipment, but my kids think it's pretty cool. The decision to live without these things reflects our family's goals and priorities, and for us, it's worked out great. Plus, I never have to argue with them to get off the computer, stop watching TV and get some exercise. They have no choice!

Each family needs to make good decisions that will reflect their own family's priorities and goals, and no one else's. And if getting exercise is part of the program, those sedentary activities such as TV watching, Nintendo and computer games may need to be scaled back. Remember, the real change will happen when real change is made.

It is here where I wish I could end this chapter, but that is impossible. I hinted about eating disorders briefly in the second chapter, but I feel it necessary to expand a bit. When I was nutritionally counseling families, I also counseled women at an upscale, trendy gym. It worked out great—I had a free membership and my nutrition clients paid me. Before the initial appointment, I had all new clients fill out nutritional questionnaires so I could review their histories. Eight out of ten of these women had either had, or was struggling with, an eating disorder. That made my jaw drop, but the thing that really blew my mind was they were all coming to me to lose weight! None of them were interested in being healthy, feeling better or having more energy as a primary goal. And every one of these clients that had an eating disorder, past or present, was dealing with health issues because of these disorders. Yet still, they wanted to lose weight. They wanted to lose that last five pounds so they wouldn't be "so horribly obese." Of course, they never were to begin with. Yet, they wanted me to put them on a new regimen to deal with these imaginary weight problems. At this time, the no-fat, high-carb diet was chi-chi and this idea of balance was horrifying and met with a lot of skepticism.

I'll never forget the one woman I sat and argued with for over an hour on why she needed to add oil in her diet. She head leathery, dry skin and didn't need to lose on ounce of fat and yet, walked out the door and I never saw her again.

Anorexia nervosa, the no-eating or almost-no-eating disorder, if allowed to run its full course, ends in death. Bulimia, the eating disorder of an estimated five million Americans, is characterized by out of control eating, followed by induced vomiting and/or the use of laxatives to avoid weight gain. Bulimia can lead to serious health issues such as ulcers, a ruptured stomach, kidney damage, erratic heartbeat, as well as ruined teeth and a psychological scar that can last a lifetime.

All eating disorders are symptoms that all is not well. The only course of action is professional intervention with an all-out focus on getting the child well. There are many different treatment programs and professionals out there, and some are better than others. It is always wise to do some serious investigation and ask some well-thought out, intelligent questions with anyone who may be treating your child for an eating disorder. There is no excuse not to have an excellent body of knowledge and understanding of what you're dealing with, especially in this day and age. Caring Online (www.caring online.com) offers comprehensive lists of symptoms, treatment facilities, news, articles and more.

Do your child a favor and become the best-educated advocate she could possibly have, your child's very life may be at stake.

CHAPTER SIX

Allergies and Your Child

The amount of alternative information available on food allergies has come a long way. There was a time when books had to be specially ordered from obscure publishers, there was no internet, and everything I'm talking about was never spoken of in front of the family doctor. We've come a long way, baby. Each stride toward true wellness has been worth the struggle in the "mainstream" medical community. A wholehearted endorsement of treating food allergies yourself as a first plan-of-attack, may never come carte blanche from the medical community. But at least there is a beginning of understanding coming from allopathic doctors that natural and logical ways of looking at health issues isn't a threat to their livelihoods.

Make no mistake about it, I have great respect for physicians, especially doctors who are able to look beyond their own comfort zones, if you will, and see the contribution that nutrition has on wellness or illness. Some experts have come to the conclusion that six out of 10 children are allergic to milk protein.

Milk and dairy products are not the sole producers of food allergies. Some other offenders may be tomatoes, corn, wheat, peanuts, soybeans, eggs or citrus, to name a few. If you suspect allergy problems with your child, it may be wise to keep a food diary of everything your child consumes; when he eats it and a comment on his reaction—bad mood, dark circles, stomach ache, etc. After a few days or weeks of doing this, you may uncover a pattern, be able to eliminate the offender and move on. Always start with taking dairy out first, as this is the most common allergen. Give it at least four weeks and see how your child does. If there is no improvement, move on to the next thing. Obviously, any child under the care of a doctor should continue to stay under a doctor's care. I am speaking to parents who may suspect their child is allergic to something and would like to do a little investigative snooping to see if they are able to uncover something.

To prevent allergies, it's best to start young. The longer your child is on the breast, the better. I am also a firm believer in delaying the introduction to solids as long as possible. However, some babies are just plain hungry and will try and eat whatever you're eating—I had one of those, too. If that is the case, make sure you give one food at a time for at least a week before introducing something new. In other words, breakfast, lunch and dinner should be green beans, if that's the food for the week. Don't skip this important step—it's easier to figure out what the allergen is when there isn't much to choose from.

ALLERGY SYMPTOMS

- Constant runny nose
- Ear infections
- Mouth breathing
- Rashes
- Eczema
- Dark circles under eyes
- Pale puffy face
- Spots on the tongue
- Stomach aches
- Constipation or diarrhea
- Irritability

Diet is so important when trying to determine the root cause of allergies. The Feingold diet, a rotation diet that eliminates allergens, has a website that offers support, help and resources. I would certainly recommend anyone who needs help, to log on to the site at www.feingold.com.

Doris Rapp, M.D. wrote an eye-opening book several years ago called, *Is This Your Child?* She showed the correlation between allergies, learning disorders and how to treat the problems naturally with a rotation diet. Doris Rapp is a hero in my eyes, and many others, too. She also has a website that is very helpful: www.dorisrapp.com.

A final note: allergies are the result of a weakened immune system. Keeping the immune system strong with good nutrition, adequate hydration, supplements and a little exercise can help make a huge difference. If you are struggling with allergies in your family, there is a lot of help available. Get yourself an education and become proactive. Even if this is all brand new to you, take heart: I am not the only one who has been there—you may yet have your own elevator experience.

PART THREE

Making Mealtime Manageable

CHAPTER SEVEN

Mealtime Mechanics

It has been said that insanity is doing the same thing over and over again and expecting different results. So why do I still think my open refrigerator door is going to suddenly inspire me with gourmet thoughts and tasty dreams for this Tuesday night dinner? Isn't it evident that it's almost time to panic? The chicken is as frozen as an igloo in Antarctica and there is no way that the ground round will thaw anytime before Spring. What's a woman to do?

The natives are restless and are beginning to circle the cat. I better do something quick. Hungry?! What do you mean you're hungry? It's only 5:45—get a grip! No one decent eats before 6:00. Maybe if I go and open the refrigerator door again, inspiration will strike.

But what is this? What doth my eye spy lurking there in the dark recesses of the freezer? To my complete and utter joy, there are approximately three tater tots and five fish sticks at the very back, trying to strike out on their own. Make that four tater tots—what looked like a brown ice cube is actually a tater tot completely encased in its own ice tomb. If I promise them ice cream for dessert, do you think this will be enough?

The tater tot is stuck to the freezer rack and comes apart as I try to pull it out. Back down to three tater tots. Nope, definitely not enough for two growing kids. Now what? Yikes, it's 6:00—now it's time to panic. You-know-who should be bursting in on the scene in about 15 minutes. What am I going to make? Two peanut butter and jelly sandwiches along with a banana each for the kids with a promise for ice cream cones tomorrow...if they promise not to tell a soul their mother, the cookbook writer, is feeding them so pathetically and is fresh out of ideas (and ingredients) for dinner.

I eyeball those fish sticks and 3½ tater tots. Evil thoughts fill my mind as I whip out the can opener and make a unique casserole, just for you-know-who. A fish stick here, a tater tot there, some Y2K cream of chicken soup in the middle, sprinkle with tarragon, top with cheese and garnish with the half a tater tot rescued from ice...I'm a genius! And as Martha would say, it's a good thing.

Sitting down to dinner as a family has almost become the exception and not the rule anymore. The family table has been sacrificed for various activities and the results are disheartening. Many families feel disconnected from each other, children are incommunicative and the opportunity to really know and care about each other is gone in the quest to get to soccer practice on time.

A little thing like trying to sit down together as a family for dinner every night, will have an impact on the family like almost nothing else. For a lot of families, this could be the only time in the day possible to in-

MOM'S SUPER HAT TRICK #1

The Taming of the Shrew

Sometimes trying a new food, can be more trying on a parent then on a child, if you get my drift. There are times when food needs to be an adventure. Not everyday, but just especially when introducing something new, especially to the little guys. Here is a great trick for presenting a food to your child.

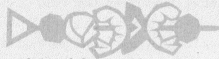

The On-A-Stick Trick

"I've got the world on a string..." so the old song goes. But if you're a kid, you could probably care less about the world being on a string or this old song. Now, if you had the world-on-a-stick, well, that's completely different.

Kids will eat anything if they get to poke it with a stick. At least one bite, anyway. Cut everything up, put it on a plate (not touching!) and give them a big toothpick. Give them a rule or two, like don't put the toothpick in your sister's eye, refrain from putting the toothpick in your ear—things like that. Then let them go to town! They'll have a blast and may actually try something they wouldn't have tried before.

You can also serve it kabob-style already stuck on a stick. That's fun too, but getting to actually skewer the food themselves is great entertainment.

teract and connect. Giving that time up to activities will undermine a family's cohesiveness. Think about it. If you don't have time to be together, you can't expect your family to be close and loving. It won't happen unless there is that investment of time.

So how do you revamp life to fit into this goal of sitting down to dinner together as a family? Let's take a hypothetical family, the Busbees (dad, mom and 2.5 kids—typical American family) and see if you can relate to their schedule. They have been complaining about the lack of family togetherness and when the family dinner table was suggested, they thought it sounded great. But the question is, for whom?

Betty Busbee, the mom, has a minivan with a bumper sticker that says "If I am a stay-at-home mom, why am I always in the car?" Naturally, she volunteers in both kids' classrooms. In addition, she teaches Sunday school, manages the family's finances, and does all the cooking and cleaning. She's also a homework helper to both kids and the captain of the phone chain for school. She does all of that in between her time in the car where she takes the kids to music lessons, band practice, ballet, tap, clogging, gymnastics, 4-H, cub scouts, girl scouts, choir, swimming lessons, swim team, soccer, baseball, volleyball and croquet.

And now, with her hair standing on end and a mad dog glint in her eyes, she asks, *"You want me to do what?"* Clearly, this is a woman who needs a break. This is a family that needs to realign their priorities.

How is this done, anyway? How can a busy Busbee family get a grip on what's important to them as a family? It starts with just that question: what is important to our family? And is what we are doing accomplishing our goals?

Let's take a look at the Busbees. For starters, Mr. and Mrs. Busbee can set down some hard and fast rules: one activity each for the kids. That can even be cinched up a little tighter to make sure that the kid's different activities are on the same day. I use that tactic a lot to keep my schedule from flying out of control, and I only have two kids! How much more important this rule is when there are more children in the home. I have one day a week that the kids have music lessons, we go to a convalescent home, and do all the errands—sort of stacking the day with all the run around stuff, rather than scattering it all out all over the week. It works well for us and helps us keep our priorities straight. You want your home to be more of a home and less of drop off point or launch pad. There's no place like home is in real danger of becoming, there is no place that's home.

The other thing the Busbees can do is not sweat the small stuff. Let's say dinner together is impossible a couple of nights a week. Have breakfast together if you can't do dinner, even if it means getting up a little earlier than normal. The important thing is sitting down together. On the other hand, it may be impossible to sit down before 7:00 pm for dinner. I am unaware of any rules that say dinner must always be eaten at 6:00. Flexibility is what will make this work.

I have reworked my schedule so that my children are a part of the dinnertime preparation and routine. This is one more way to develop good relationships with your children. Both of my children look forward to their turn when they get to be mom's kitchen helper. My daughter, though just 10, can already make burritos, scrambled eggs, pancakes and bake cookies, and makes lunch for her brother and me regularly. She can easily clean up a kitchen single-handedly. She has learned to do these things by my side as my kitchen helper. My eight-year-old son is an expert carrot and potato peeler, pancake turner over-er, and terrific salad maker. And he has learned to dry and put away dishes, sweep and wipe down the counters and table. If something needs vacuuming, I call in the expert, my son.

The point is when children have a vested interest in helping the family reach its goal of drawing closer, they pitch in and do what they can to help. If the burden is all on mom's shoulders to do all the cleaning, cooking and cleaning up, she's overworked, overburdened and what should be a relaxing, enjoyable time is just another thing on her list of things to do. Not only will these trained and efficient kitchen and household helpers make a difference at home, they're having an opportunity to exercise their work ethic at an early age—something that will serve them and their employer well when they get older. This all works in tandem with the idea that as the workload is spread out, the family has more time together. Everyone is happier, especially mom!

Once you finally do get to the sitting down together part, enjoy each other! Don't rush through dinner and start barking orders to get the table cleared. Sit and savor the moment. Laugh at your preschoolers silly joke told for the fiftieth time, listen intently as your son talks about catching that fly ball. By giving your children eye contact and truly listening, they know they are

MOM'S SUPER HAT TRICK #2

With-A-Dip

You want to increase your chances that your child will actually like the new food? That he will actually eat the new food? Try it on-a-stick, try it with-a-dip.

Will he eat it with a dip? Will he eat it on a chip?

Does he like this new food taste? Or will this squash just go to waste?

It can be downright depressing trying to expand a younger child's repetoire. But not when you can whip out a stick and bring on the dip!

The dip factor is an old trick, but unfortunately, many parents are tempted to give kids ketchup on everything or bury the vegetables in icky ranch dressing. Check out the dips in the recipe section for some other ideas. And then keep a lot on hand!

loved and cared about. Good healthy food on their plates can never take the place of a parent who is truly there with their child, in the moment, listening to their stories, complaints and goofball jokes.

But where was dad in all this dinner preparation? Why scrubbing the toilet bowl, of course. Actually, the real reason I didn't include him in this dinner time scheme is because for us, he's usually arriving after all the action has taken place. And I've found that's the case with a lot of families. But that doesn't mean Mr. Wonderful gets the best spot on the couch and full remote privileges. Helping to clean up or taking the kids for a while after dinner, offers great time for dad and kids to reconnect. Nothing will cause a woman to get more resentful quicker than having a hubby come home and get comatose on the couch after dinner. There are still dishes to do, children to be bathed, stories to be read. So even if your husband misses all the preparation for dinner, he can still be a big part of this new and improved plan of family togetherness. His participation is as important as everyone else's.

All of this will help create a family identity and bring everyone close. I tell my kids that they are "the excellent Ely's and we do things excellently". I don't tell them this so they can proclaim themselves superior to the world, but so they'll eventually hold up high and excellent standards for themselves and their own families when they are grown. From their vantage point and ages, I'm sure my children probably don't see how any of this interrelates, but it does. Like a gigantic tapestry, all these things act like different colored threads to make one beautiful masterpiece. If all you could see was the backside of a tapestry, you would see all the work that went into making this fine piece—the knots, the patterns and continuity of color—all of the hidden work. Not too impressive, if that was all you saw. But when you turn it over, the beauty of this work will take your breath away. This is what the family dinner table represents. A constant thread in the tapestry of our family's life. While only a single thread to a bigger canvas, its interwoven pattern strengthens and clarifies the big picture on the other side. Without it, the whole thing would fall apart.

CHAPTER EIGHT

Manners for the not so Mannerly

Turn away when spitting lest your saliva fall on someone. If anything purulent falls on the ground, it should be trodden upon, lest it nauseate someone.

To lick greasy fingers or to wipe them on your coat is impolite. It is better to use the tablecloth or the serviette.

Some people put their hands in the dishes the moment they have sat down. Wolves do that.

You should not offer your handkerchief to anyone unless it has been freshly washed. Nor is it seemly, after wiping your nose, to spread out your handkerchief and peer into it as if pearl and rubies might have fallen out of your head.

Retain the wind by compressing the belly.

Do not be afraid of vomiting, if you must; for it is not vomiting but holding the vomit in your throat that is foul.

If you cannot swallow a piece of food, turn around discreetly and throw it somewhere.

Do not move back and forth on your chair. Whoever does that give the impression of constantly breaking or trying to break wind.

We have Erasmus (c.1530) to thank for these fine etiquette tips. Of course, a few things have changed in these last 400 plus years, rest assured.

Or have they? Etiquette experts from Miss Manners to Emily Post bemoan our seemingly barbaric manners at the table as they try to answer, as mannerly as possible, the etiquette questions they are asked by a less than civilized culture. Our manners seem to have taken a leave of absence.

Pushing food onto forks with fingers, slurping, belching and talking on cell phones at the table is an abominable sight to behold. But a sight to behold nonetheless. Next time you are in a restaurant, look for yourself. These are the adults—the children are worse.

The dinner table at home is even less sacrosanct—if there is even a table being eaten around. Children today are growing up wiping their mouths on their sleeves and putting such large forkfuls of food in their mouths, that for a parent, knowing the Heimlich manuever is essential.

To grow up and not know how to eat politely will become a social barrier for the untrained. Rebecca Bruce, president and chief executive of Aon Management Institute of Glastonbury, Michigan has made her life's work etiquette and the teaching of table manners. Being unlearned herself, this deficit in her upbringing caused her to commit social hari-kari at an important business dinner, when she mistakenly ate the dinner roll off her boss' plate. "He pointed it out to me," she said, the memory obviously permanently etched in her mind. "A person lacking in table graces is absolutely at a disadvantage. A person may have all the technical skills, but unless they're able to represent the company in social situations, they will never be asked to attend meetings with higher executives. Once you know table manners, it is second nature and you're so much more comfortable," she said.

I can relate. Dinnertime at my house has very little in common with those wonderful Norman Rockwell pictures you see of a family around the dinner table. The most obvious missing element would be the mom in the June Cleaver look-alike outfit—sweats from Wal-Mart are more my speed. But take a good look at the children in those pictures—they eat with their mouths closed—you can't see the child's tonsils and spaghetti at the same time.

When we bow our heads at the dinner table, I silently offer up my own plea to God for some manners from the children. I ask God to help my children speak without a chicken leg taking up the space between their teeth and cheek. I beg Him to help my children see that eating a piece of pot roast the size of a gerbil could prove hazardous. And lastly, I ask Him, if all of the above fails, please give me grace to remind them again about their manners with a little dignity. Throwing myself on the floor and begging is downright humiliating.

And speaking of dinner tables—unless you happen to have a Hoover-ish dog in the family, who uses the space under the dinner table as a buffet line—there seems to be more dinner allotted to the floor, than to the kids. Why is that? Is the food problematic?

Let's take a look at tonight's dinner, for example: meatloaf, check. Mashed potatoes, check. Broccoli, cut into bite sized pieces, no less, check. Seems like a simple meal to get onto one's fork and into one's mouth, right? No rolling, wayward peas or long, slippery pasta on my table. Just simple, forkable food. But in-between the fork and mouth is that deep chasm—the dining room floor. And it is there where meatloaf, broccoli and mashed potatoes congregate on a nightly basis, until a foot puts them in their place: smashed into the area rug.

If I could have a drain in the middle of my dining room floor and a fire hose attachment in the kitchen, I might not complain so much. But sadly, that is not the case, although I am thankful for wood floors. They're a little more forgiving, if you're smarter than I am and skip the antique hook rug under the table.

So how do we bring up these children of ours to not be social misfits and ne'er-do-wells at the dinner table? In the end, I found the real answer to decent table manners, more often than not, lies with the parents. Children must be trained and part of that training is from example. Here are few dinner table rules to consider for everyone involved:

Put your napkin on your lap. It requires very little energy to do so and will endear you forever to the hostess.

Wait for the blessing, if one is said. If you want to blow away the hostess, wait for her to sit down and pick up her fork.

Manage unchewables wisely. If you find you must spit something out, it is better to use your napkin than to gross out the entire table with the big wad of unchewable meat you pulled out with your hands and perched on the side of your plate. It is also unnecessary to make an announcement about your finding.

Stop the slurp. If you are drinking something from a glass or enjoying your soup, it is preferable to do so silently. It is unnerving to well-mannered guests to listen to five people at the same time slurp soup.

Don't fetch. It is better to ask your table mate to pass something to you, than reach across him and drag your sleeve through his gravy. This will most assuredly cause great distress to the person whose plate you have desecrated and the person in charge of laundry.

Common courtesies. The words "please" and "thank-you" have not been stricken from the English language. Use them liberally.

Dental dispatch. If there is something big and green stuck in someone's teeth at the table, make inconspicuous hand gestures to notify him or her. Again, loud announcements of this sort are completely unnecessary. Likewise, if there is something big and green stuck in your teeth and someone gestures to you about it, kindly ask to be excused and take care of it out of view.

Using a fork tine, credit card or even toothpick to dislodge the intruder at the table is highly frowned upon.

For some reason, manners aren't taught as quickly as they are caught. Becoming vigilant with dinner table habits will serve everyone well in the family. Manners are a common ground that help to establish the dinner table as an enjoyable place to be. Use them, and they will serve you. Forget about them, and they (or the lack of them) will embarrass you. It is a simple thing that costs nothing and yet could cost everything.

Manners are essential: don't leave home without them.

CHAPTER NINE

A Good Cook Cooks

This tendency toward convenience foods is rather distressing. True, it is helpful to have something to pull out of your hat when you need to fly out the door for baseball practice, but it doesn't have to come in a box from the freezer and go into the microwave. There is a better solution.

Everything in life worth something has taken some effort. This is also true with trying to eat healthier. It will require some effort on your part, but with a little bit of forethought and a few good moves, it won't be too hard. Plus, I would never leave a mom in the lurch without one or two quick tricks—we all need them, don't we?

So let's start in the kitchen. I have a few good tools I wouldn't want to be without. And then I have some real time saving tools, I call my indentured servants because these babies make life a little easier.

Here's the list:

Good, sharp knives—a dull knife will make tomato sauce out of your tomatoes. It is a joy to work with a good knife. I have had my Henckle chef knife for over 20 years and it's just as wonderful as the first day I bought it. Good knives are a great tool, if they are kept sharpened.

A few cutting boards—working with just one cutting board is a mistake. With all the scary information out there on salmonella and the rest, it might not be a bad idea to be a little more kosher about your cutting boards: use one for vegetables, fruit etc. and one ONLY for meat.

A flat-bottomed wok—another tool I have owned for a long time. This stainless, well-seasoned pan has scrambled eggs and cooked countless stir frys. I truly wouldn't be without it, and the flat-bottom is essential—no fussing with a ring and a wobbly pan on the stove.

Vegetable steamer—Unless you forget about your vegetables in the steamer, you almost can't wreck them. Plus, they're never soggy.

Popsicle molds—cheap and easy dessert for your kids and you, for that matter. Buy them when you see them and buy a couple of sets. Good luck finding them in the middle of January, however.

Stainless or non-aluminum cookware—aluminum has been linked to all kinds of health problems, and rather than debate the issue, why not just get some decent stainless steel pots and pans and forget about it?

Cupcake liners. I don't know why on earth it took

me so long to figure out that cupcake liners can be used for muffins, too. I have seen them used that way in bakery muffins, but I guess I'm just a slow learner. Cupcake liners keep clean up to a minimum and really simplify the process.

A stash of Pyrex dishes that you can fill and throw in your freezer. If you can get in the habit of doubling your family's dinner, you can stock a mother lode of meals in the freezer with very little extra effort.

A timer. If you are anything like me, your good intentions can turn into burnt offerings. A good working timer with a buzzer you can actually hear is a smart choice.

A quality wire whisk. There is nothing better than a good whisk for beating eggs, making sauces, gravies, etc. An unbeatable have-to-have tool.

Microwave, for quick heat ups, not cooking.

Pizza stone (good bye Pizza parlors!)

Now, bring on the servants! These appliances need to be seen with new eyes.

That isn't just a crockpot hiding in the dark corners of your cupboard. That's a cook who'll be whipping up something fabulous for you and your family while you're running around all day or at work. Do you see why you need to yank that thing out from the netherworld of your cupboard?

And the bread machine you got as an anniversary present or wedding gift? Your own personal baker! The freezer? A virtual restaurant waiting to be heated up. Your food processor? Your own personal kitchen assistant.

What more could a gal ask for? Every one of these tools gets neglected from time to time, but if you use them, you'll find yourself able to do so much more in the kitchen and it will be so much easier to cook. With a little bit of planning, some good recipes (got 'em right here!) and a willingness to try something new, your kitchen will never be the same.

Pantry Basics

I have said it before, I'll say it again, a well-stocked pantry is a gal's best friend. Not having to duck out to the grocery store just to get dinner on the table is wonderful. Living that way on a day in-day out basis is glorious. I wouldn't exaggerate about such things.

Pantries can either be full of a bunch of stuff you'll never use—like hearts of palm and creamed corn buried in the dark corners or full of things you use constantly. If you're good at stocking your pantry, the only thing you'll need to concern yourself with is rotating your stock (yep, just like a grocery store!)

For newbie pantry stockers, there is an answer and there is hope. Here I come to save the day! It's Healthy Mom to the rescue! I have some basics for you right here in these next few pages. We are talking about healthy stuff here, but understand something also. I am not made out of endless amounts of cash and don't spend frivolously. Even if I were, I wouldn't. So take your time stocking your pantry, look for specials and sales and *then* go crazy buying canned tomatoes.

If you are living in tight quarters and feel you can't afford a pantry, start a massive decluttering plan and start looking. If you're smart and creative, you can always pull a rabbit out of your hat. During the Y2K madness, (okay, I'll admit it!) I had cases of canned goods under my bed, the kids beds and dressers. I pulled stuff out and rotated with stuff from the cupboards. So it wasn't the most convenient. It worked, though.

Stocking the Pantry

An important aspect of being able to plan and cook efficiently has to do with what Amy Dacyczyn, the author of *The Tightwad Gazette* calls The Pantry Principle. The idea behind the Pantry Principle is to stockpile your basics for your pantry so you don't run out. And you do this buying only on sale, with a coupon or at a salvage/scratch and dent-type store. The Pantry Principle liberated me from rigid menu planners, last minute trips to the grocery store, and the best part is that it kept my budget in line.

The Pantry Principle gives you the freedom to plan your meals around what's in your pantry, so that when you do your grocery shopping, you are actually shopping to replenish pantry supplies and not buying a bunch of stuff just for specific meals.

While everyone's pantry might look a little different, here's what's in my pantry and what I would suggest you might want to include in yours, especially if you're going to make any of the recipes in this book! Remember to use the Pantry Principle as you plan your grocery shopping. Never having to run to the store for one or two ingredients because of your principled pantry, is a gift of time that you give yourself that is even more valuable than the money saved.

BAKING SUPPLIES:

Baking powder (look for one without aluminum sulfate. Try the health food store and remember to refrigerate to keep it fresh!)

Baking soda

Sea salt

Cocoa or **carob** (*I have cocoa—see glossary for explanation*)

Vinegars: rice wine, red wine, balsamic, apple cider

Whole wheat flour*

Whole wheat pastry flour* (*see glossary for explanation on the differences in flour*)

Gluten*(*helps make bread rise better*)

Kamut flour

Whole oats*

Buckwheat flour*

Cornmeal *

Whole grain pancake mix*

Sucanat (*see glossary*)

Unsulphured molasses

Pure vanilla extract

*From the bulk bins at the health food store. I keep mine in plastic containers with screw on tops

BREADS:

Whole wheat bread

Rye bread
Tortillas: sprouted whole wheat (health food store), corn
Bagels

CANNED GOODS:
Tomato puree
Diced tomatoes
Whole stewed tomatoes
Tomato paste
Pumpkin puree
Pineapple
Apple sauce (although I make it, I like to have it on hand, too)
Evaporated milk
Tuna
Green chilies
Beans (an assortment for emergencies, otherwise I make my own)
Salsas
Pickles (an assortment, plus what I've canned—zucchini relish, okra pickles, pickle pickles)

CONDIMENTS:
Soy sauce
Sesame oil
Ketchup
Mustards (regular yellow, dijon, honey mustard, coarse)
Honey *
Jams (raspberry, wild blackberry, plum and peach that I canned)
Peanut butter
Almond butter*
Tahini (see glossary)

SEASONINGS:
Peppercorns (use a grinder and grind your own. A quantum leap above the already ground stuff)
Nutmeg nuts (I bought some at a dollar store and the itty, bitty grater came with it—unbeatable flavor)
Ground nutmeg (only get this if you can't find nutmeg nuts and the itty, bitty grater)
Garlic powder (NOT salt)
Tarragon
Rosemary
Bay leaves
Basil
Sage
Thyme
Ginger
Cloves
Mace
Curry powder
Paul Prudhomme's Pasta & Pizza seasoning (a little pricey, but so good)

CEREALS:
Wheat chex
Cheerios
Kamut flakes
Whole oats
7 grain cereal
Puffed wheat, millet, kamut, brown rice
Ancient Grains Cereals (President's Choice brand—widely available in supermarkets everywhere)

PREPACKAGED STUFF:
White macaroni and cheese (*no junky food colorings*)

LEGUMES & GRAINS & PASTA:
Barley (*not pearled*)
Split peas
Lentils
Black beans
Turtle beans
Pintos
White beans
Navy beans
Brown rice (*short and long grain*)
Brown basmati rice
Cous cous
Kamut pastas (*we like this better than whole wheat*)

PANTRY VEGGIES:
Potatoes
Onions
Sweet potatoes
Garlic
Assorted winter squashes when in season

REFRIGERATOR:
Milk
Butter
Eggs
Cheeses (*romano, cheddar, jack—block and shredded*)
Tofu
Yogurt (*homemade or store bought*)
Cold-pressed oils (*I have olive oil and safflower*)

Flax seeds
Yeast
Mayonnaise
Worcestershire sauce (*probably not necessary to refrigerate, but I do*)

FREEZER:
Chicken
Beef
Frozen vegetables (*for emergency dinners, otherwise I use fresh and in-season*)
Frozen fruits (*for smoothies*)
Frozen overripe bananas (*ditto*)
Orange juice
Cheeses
Butter
Homemade popcicles

FRUIT BASKET:
Apples
Bananas

VEGETABLE BIN:
Carrots
Celery

Other than that, whatever I have—either grown or bought from a veggie stand or on sale at the market. I only buy in-season fruit and vegetables, with the exception of apples, onions, bananas and potatoes.

The Efficient Kitchen

You can have all the latest and greatest tools, indentured servants and principled pantries in the world and you still won't have an efficient kitchen. Efficient kitchens are implemented by doing something with them. They don't just happen on their own.

To make this happen, you need a plan. Not a great big, complicated system that requires tickler cards, menu planning galore and a day off from life to figure it out. Some simple strategies, a few well-thought out rules—and bingo, you have efficiency.

First things first. Dinner. Believe it or not, there are a lot of people out there who don't even think about dinner till around 4:00. Or till they are driving home from work. Regardless, this is a poor strategy, or really a non-strategy because the results are always the same: either a late dinner, a microwaved dinner, or fast food.

Awhile back, when I was doing a time management seminar with my friend Demaris Ford (one of the tasters in the cookbook section), she introduced the Ten O'clock Principle. The Ten O'clock Principle is simply, that you decide on your dinner each night by 10:00 that morning. However, if you know that Wednesday, for example, is always very busy, then you decide on dinner for Wednesday night on Tuesday night at 10:00 PM. The Ten O'Clock Principle is the same, you just move it around (AM or PM) accordingly. That way, you can prepare! Like take something out of the freezer to thaw, plug something into the indentured servant (crockpot) or check to make sure you have charcoal for the barbeque. While this is a great concept for many families, I have simplified it even further for my own family.

Monday—spaghetti or lasagna

Tuesday—Breakfast for dinner

Wednesday—crockpot chili (or something crock potty)

Thursday—salad and sandwich supper

Friday—Rubber chicken* *(see recipe section)*

Saturday—chicken burritos or another selection using leftover chicken

Sunday—a chicken stock-based soup

Vegetables and/or plenty of salad is usually served with every meal, except Breakfast for dinner.

I did this because I basically didn't want to think about it. This schedule still allows me plenty of creativity, and though we don't rigidly follow it, I like the idea of being able to say, "It's Monday, so we're having spaghetti tonight." This summer, we had lots of squash and tomatoes given to us and we grew our own green beans and corn. So we enjoyed the bounty with a vegetable supper and some homemade cornbread or whole grain bread.

Another efficient thing to do is make double or even triple dinner. You can freeze a meal, and put some in the fridge for leftovers. We eat leftover dinner 9 times out of 10 the next day for lunch. Makes lunch time a snap and I appreciate the time off from having to constantly engage my brain. Sometimes the question about what the next meal is can send me into a downward spiral. Every little bit helps, you know.

Family-Tested Recipes

Breakfast in Bread

& Other Comforts

There's plenty here to start your morning off right. Breakfast will never be the same if you try a couple of new recipes. Just make sure you double or even triple some of the muffin recipes—they're too good not to have a few tucked in the freezer.

And if you're after breakfast-in-a-glass, these smoothies will knock your socks off.

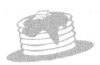

Apricot Oatbran Muffins

I experimented for a long time with this recipe. I really wanted a lot of fiber in them, but they started to taste like I dumped sawdust in them or something. Muffins shouldn't be that fibrous. I think these ones are good without being too woody, if you know what I mean. Makes a dozen.

1 cup oat bran

1 ½ cups whole wheat pastry flour

¼ cup organic sucanat

1 tablespoon baking powder

2 egg whites, or whole eggs

1 cup skim milk, make sour with 1 teaspoon vinegar (or use buttermilk)

1 teaspoon vanilla extract

¼ cup safflower oil, or Better Butter (pg. 150) or butter

1 jar apricot baby food or use same amount of fruit sweetened apricot preserves

1/8 teaspoon sea salt

Preheat oven to 350 degrees. Prepare muffin tin by either greasing or using cupcake liners.

In a large bowl, mix together dry ingredients and make a well in the center. In a separate bowl, mix wet ingredients well and add to dry ingredients. Mix till combined, but don't overdo it.

Spoon batter into prepared muffin tin, filling each cup ¾ full.

Bake for 18-20 minutes. Cool for 5 minutes in muffin tin, then remove individual muffins to a wire rack to cool.

PER SERVING: 95 CALORIES (KCAL); 5G TOTAL FAT; (42% CALORIES FROM FAT); 3G PROTEIN; 13G CARBOHYDRATE; TRACE CHOLESTEROL; 162MG SODIUM

"These are moist and delicious! I think the preserves give more apricot flavor than the baby food." —Marilyn May

"I really like these muffins! They have a nice flavor, and they're especially good warm with butter." —Deborah Hockman

Glossary of New Terms

Adzuki beans—I don't mention them in this book, but if you run into them, you should know what they are. Similar to a black bean, they are small red beans that are the lowest in fat of all beans.

Bok Choy—a big, vegetable thing that looks like a cross between lettuce and cabbage. Great in stir fry.

Brown rice—this is the only kind of rice to buy, although there are tons of different types of brown rice available: short grain, long grain, basmati, for example. For more on rice, see "Righteous Rice" on page 106.

Better Butter—made with half cold pressed oil and half butter, whipped and kept refrigerated in a plastic tub, it's a good option as a spread and when a recipe calls for butter.

Butter—Yes, it is a saturated fat that is lousy for your heart. But in very small quantities (especially better butter), it's okay.

Carob—fake chocolate. What can I say? Sometimes real is better.

Cumin—often used in Mexican cooking, this spice is fabulous in all sorts of roles. You can get it relatively inexpensively at discount stores now.

Expeller-pressed oils—A.K.A. cold pressed. Oils that have been pressed by means of pressure and not chemicals or heat, thereby preserving the essential fatty acids (EFA'S). ALL Cold pressed oils need to be refrigerated after opening, including olive oil. One of the healthiest things you can do is get good, cold pressed oil and keep it refrigerated.

Flax seeds—don't waste your money on flax meal. The essential fatty acids (EFA's) in it won't be worth a nickel. Buy whole seeds, keep refrigerated and grind yourself in a coffee grinder set apart for just this task. Or I use a little Cuisinart that works well for this purpose, too. Use on top of cereal, but don't cook it or good bye EFA's.

Ginger—a strange looking, alien-like root mass that has a positively intoxicating affect on your stir fry. Buy some, freeze it and pull it out to use again and again. *(See Spice Primer for using dried ginger.)*

Gluten—gross sounding name, but essential for decent bread. Gluten is what gives bread it's lightness and tenderness. You can buy bread flour (not recommended if it's white flour) or get the gluten. Found at health food stores, mostly.

Greens—if you live in the South, you know what I'm talking about, if you don't then you don't know what you're missing. Mustard greens, turnip greens, kale, collards, creasy greens—all of these will grow with ease in your garden and are delicious and very nutritious. They may be found in ethnic grocers or health food stores. Just don't fix them the way they would in the South, though. Fatback is a no-no big time. Steam well and serve with rice wine vinegar. Yummy!

Jicama—a weird looking root vegetable that sort of looks like a big brown turnip. The good thing about jicama is the crunch factor. It's sweet and good in salads or served with dip.

Kamut—this is an ancient grain, recently rediscovered. Kamut is low in gluten for gluten-intolerant folks and is wonderfully wheat-y for those who can't tolerate wheat, but would love something similar. Full of protein, more so than wheat.

Lentils—are quick cooking and absolutely delicious. It should be a crime to not eat lentil soup in the winter with homemade bread.

Margarine—the ultimate sacrilege in healthy eating. Full of trans-fatty acids, this stuff will age you as fast as going to the beach without sunscreen.

Millet—bird seed. Actually, puffed millet is a great cereal for kids. Also, dried millet is another carbohydrate option instead of rice. Our family goes for the puffed variety. The parakeet is into the dried.

Miso—this is a fermented paste made out of soybeans. Even though it looks like paste wax for your car, it can sure add some body to a weak soup, or make a good soup all by itself with some sliced green onion in it, like at the sushi bar.

Maple syrup—buy the kind that comes from the tree, not the one with a log cabin or a smiling lady on the bottle. It's expensive, but it's real. I get mine at Sam's Club where it is a lot cheaper and mix it with a little bit of unsulphured molasses and honey. That stretches it a bit.

Pastry Flour—the whole wheat variety, of course. A gentler, kinder wheat with less gluten than whole wheat, this is an excellent flour for cookies, pies, cakes and muffins.

Quinoa—(keen-wa) yet another ancient grain, highest amount of protein in a grain. Try it instead of rice, made like a pilaf. (There is even a recipe right here in this book for you to try!)

Rice Milk—a milk substitute made from rice. My son drank this by the case as a toddler. Great for milk allergy folks.

Sea salt—much better than commercial salt, there are more trace minerals and less sodium chloride than regular table salt.

Sesame oil—don't forget about this wonderful oil when you're making stir fry. Toasted sesame oil is strong so you only need a little.

Soy Milk—an alternative to cow's milk, this is great for allergic folks, both in cooking and on cereal. Lots of different brands and even flavors. You need to try some out to determine which one works for you.

Spelt—another ancient grain that is great for wheat sensitive folks. A nuttier flavor, and slightly heavier, it makes good bread.

Sprouts—There are lots of sprouts out there that are wonderful on salads, sandwiches and cooked in stir fry. I love radish sprouts on sandwiches, my kids beg for a broccoli/mustard sprout blend when we go to the store, and of course, the standard mung bean sprouts are always there. Just be choosy and avoid slimy sprouts like the plague.

Sucanat—stands for Sugar Cane Natural—get it? This is evaporated sugar cane juice. Use like sugar, it's a great healthy substitute.

Tahini—like peanut butter, only made from sesame seeds. Tahini makes a great salad dressing, dip and sauce.

Tofu—some people really get into tofu, but I

mainly use silkened tofu in smoothies, or regular tofu blended to substitute for ricotta in a recipe. When my kids were babies, I'd feed them chunks of this. Great toddler food, but they like really bland stuff. For more on tofu, see Tofu Tidbits on page 140.

Vinegar—balsamic is wonderful for salads, so is rice wine vinegar. Also try apple cider and red wine.

Whole wheat—the only type of wheat product you should be buying. If it doesn't say whole wheat, it's not.

Best-ever Week-end Pancakes

There ought to be a law that whoever cooks won't gain weight. These pancakes about do in any good intentions I have about staying away from too many carbs.

Serves 8

2 cups whole wheat pastry flour
2 ½ teaspoons baking powder
½ teaspoon nutmeg
½ teaspoon cinnamon
¼ teaspoon sea salt
1 ½ cups buttermilk
5 tablespoons organic sucanat
1 egg
1 egg white
2 tablespoons unsalted butter, melted and cooled

In a large bowl, toss all dry ingredients together. Make a well in the middle.

In another bowl, mix all wet ingredients well. Add to dry ingredient and mix some more.

Let the batter sit for a minute as you prepare the griddle or pan. Heat over medium high heat, lightly grease the pan and cook pancakes as usual. Serve with real maple syrup and butter.

PER SERVING: 91 CALORIES (KCAL); 4G TOTAL FAT; (37% CALORIES FROM FAT); 3G PROTEIN; 12G CARBOHYDRATE; 33MG CHOLESTEROL; 274MG SODIUM

"We all loved them and I'm not much of a pancake person. My husband asked if we could have them all the time now! (I use Kamut for my pastry flour) They were light and fluffy and very quick to make. I found them to be as quick as a boxed mix. Yum!" —Lisa Young

"A pancake is not just a pancake! These pancakes are not just delicious they are wholesome too! I couldn't help but think what a wonderful recipe to serve company, they just might want to stay longer! We like thinner batter for our pancakes so we added a little bit more buttermilk. Mmm!" —Susie

Buckwheat PannyCakes

When my kids were little, this is what they called them and the name stuck. At my age, I have no excuse for baby talk, but these fluffy pancakes beg such a childish name! You'll see why when you make them yourself.

Serves 4

1 cup whole wheat pastry flour
½ cup buckwheat flour
¼ cup organic sucanat
2 teaspoons baking powder
1 ½ cups skim milk, or buttermilk
1 tablespoon safflower oil
1 egg, you can substitute 2 egg whites if you prefer

In a large bowl, combine dry ingredients. Make a well in the center

In a smaller bowl, combine milk, egg and safflower oil. Mix well.

Pour wet into dry and mix well, but don't overdo it. If they seem a little dry, add a little more milk or water even.

Cook pancakes as usual and serve with real maple syrup and a little butter.

PER SERVING: 186 CALORIES (KCAL); 5G TOTAL FAT; (23% CALORIES FROM FAT); 6G PROTEIN; 31G CARBOHYDRATE; 48MG CHOLESTEROL; 307MG SODIUM

All four of my kids absolutely loved the Buckwheat PannyCakes! My 10-year-old daughter's response when she first tasted these was:'Mmm. These are good. It doesn't need syrup. It's sweetened already." —Bonnie Musselwhite

Buttermilk Cornbread

This is what you must make when you're having beans—no question about it.
It's as easy as making pancakes, too.
Serves 10

1 cup white cornmeal, use yellow if you
   can't find white
1 cup whole wheat pastry flour
1 ½ tablespoons sucanat
2 teaspoons baking powder
½ teaspoon baking soda
½ teaspoon sea salt
1 cup buttermilk
2 eggs, beaten

In a mixing bowl, toss together dry ingredients and make a well in the middle.

In another bowl, mix beaten eggs and buttermilk together. Stir into dry ingredients till moistened. Don't over mix unless your goal is adobe bricks. Pour batter into a greased 8" pan.

Bake in a 425 degree preheated oven for 18 to 20 minutes. Check it though...and pull it out when a toothpick inserted in the middle comes out clean.

PER SERVING: 74 CALORIES (KCAL); 1G TOTAL FAT; (16% CALORIES FROM FAT); 3G PROTEIN; 12G CARBOHYDRATE; 38MG CHOLESTEROL; 292MG SODIUM

"This cornbread is fantastic! I love the combination of bran and corn flavor. This cornbread is delicious with or without butter. It is a very quick and easy recipe."—Marilyn May

Cinna-Buns

Whole wheat bread morphing into cinnamon rolls. How'd she do that?
Serves 8

1 recipe Elise Clark's Wondrous Whole Wheat Bread, follow directions for bread, but set on dough cycle, not to bake for bread
½ cup honey, you may need a little more
½ cup nuts or raisins or ½ cut of each, optional
3 tbsp. cinnamon

When dough is done in your Automatic Bread Machine (or you could have made the bread dough according to the recipe on *page 68*), roll it out on a floured surface with your rolling pin till about ¼-½" thick. Spoon honey on to surface and evenly distribute. Generously sprinkle cinnamon and top with optional nuts and raisins. Roll up like you would a sleeping bag, then cut carefully with a serrated knife and put the pinwheel-like creations right next to each other in a lightly greased 9 X 13 pan. Bake for 15-20 minutes (depending on how big your buns are) in a 350 degree oven.

Top with cream cheese icing if you want (*see page 175*). Makes 8 Cinna-buns.

PER SERVING: 515 CALORIES (KCAL); 1G TOTAL FAT; (9.6% CALORIES FROM FAT); 1G PROTEIN; 140G CARBOHYDRATE; 0MG CHOLESTEROL; 7MG SODIUM

Cinnamon Coffee Cake Streusel Muffins

A special muffin for a special occasion…this is a little higher in fat than most, but so good!
Makes a dozen

1 ¾ cups whole wheat pastry flour
¾ cup organic sucanat
1 tablespoon baking powder
½ teaspoon ground cinnamon
2 egg whites
2/3 cup buttermilk
¼ cup safflower oil
1 teaspoon vanilla extract
Topping
1/8 cup unsalted butter
½ cup oats
¼ cup organic sucanat

Preheat oven to 375 degrees and prepare muffin tin by either greasing or using cupcake liners

In a large bowl, blend all dry ingredients and make a well in the middle.

In a smaller bowl, mix wet ingredients. Make streusel topping by blending butter, oats and organic sucanat till crumbly. Set aside.

Mix wet ingredients into dry ingredients till combined, but don't over do it.

Spoon the batter into a prepared muffin tin and top with streusel topping.

Bake for 15-20 minutes. Cool in pan for 5 minutes, then transfer to a rack till cooled.

PER SERVING: 167 CALORIES (KCAL); 7G TOTAL FAT; (36% CALORIES FROM FAT); 2G PROTEIN; 25G CARBOHYDRATE; 6MG CHOLESTEROL; 146MG SODIUM

"These have a wonderful taste. I'm going to make it as a coffee cake next time and save a couple of minutes Make sure you don't fill your muffin cups too full—or these will fall."—Marcella Burns

Crockpot Cereal

The recipe here is more a timesaving device than a recipe. Just follow the directions on any hot cereal you have. Measurement for one serving—multiply it to fit your family.

2/3 cup dry uncooked cereal, like oats, 7 grain, etc.
1 ½ cups water
1 tablespoon flax seeds, ground
sucanat or honey

Put on low in your crockpot overnight...that's all.

In the morning, serve into each individual bowl and top with freshly ground flax seeds. Flax seeds taste kind of nutty, and add a lot of EFA's to your bowl. Remember, *never* cook flax or you lose your EFA's!

PER SERVING: 48 CALORIES (KCAL); 3G TOTAL FAT; (58% CALORIES FROM FAT); 2G PROTEIN; 3G CARBOHYDRATE; 0MG CHOLESTEROL; 14MG SODIUM

"A fast, easy way to have a hot breakfast ready on rushed mornings. So simple, yet delicious." —Christina Fredricks

Elise Clark's Wondrous Whole Wheat Bread

I have no idea where Elise is anymore, but this is her recipe—she deserves the credit. And of all the whole wheat bread recipes out there, this is still my favorite.

Makes one loaf

1 cup + 2 tablespoons water
2 tablespoons unsalted butter or use oil
2 tablespoons honey
2 teaspoons yeast
1 ½ teaspoons sea salt
3 cups whole wheat flour
3 tablespoons gluten

Put these ingredients in your ABM the way they are listed, unless your ABM's manual wants you to put dry ingredients first. Then just reverse the list and put the last one first and continue bottom to top on the list, adding them that way...make sense?

Select your bread choice and color of crust—or however it works with your ABM, and then (my favorite part) Push Start! That's it!

PER SERVING: 131 CALORIES (KCAL); 3G TOTAL FAT; (16% CALORIES FROM FAT); 4G PROTEIN; 25G CARBOHYDRATE; 5MG CHOLESTEROL; 238MG SODIUM

COOKING NOTES: I have slightly adapted this for one of my favorite indentured servants, the ABM. Also known as, the Automatic Bread Machine. I have also noticed that with ABM's, that little bit of gluten makes a difference in the rise, although you could certainly make it without it. I am sure there is someone out there that likes doing bread completely by hand, but I'm not one of them!

Non Bread Machine Instructions for Making Bread:

Dissolve yeast in ½ cup warm water in large mixing bowl. Stir in honey, butter, salt, warm water and the whole wheat flour. Beat until smooth. Mix in enough flour to make dough easy to handle.

Turn your dough onto a lightly oiled surface: knead until smooth and elastic, about 10 minutes. Place in a greased bowl; turn greased side up. Cover; let rise in warm place until doubled, about 1 hour. (Dough is ready if an indentation remains when touched.)

Punch down dough; divide into halves. Flatten each half with your hands. Fold crosswise into thirds, overlapping the two sides. Roll up tightly, beginning at one of the open ends. Press with thumbs to seal after each turn. Pinch edge firmly to seal. Press each end with the side of your hand to seal it; fold ends under loaf. Place loaves, seam side down, in two greased loaf pans (9x3). Let rise until doubled, about one hour.

Heat oven to 375 degrees. Bake until loaves are golden brown for 40 to 45 minutes. Remove from pans; cool on wire rack. I put a clean tea towel over the top to prevent the crust from getting too hard.

Yeast—Don't be intimidated!

My friend Falinda has some friends she calls her "little red hen friends". They grow the wheat, they pick the wheat, they grind it, knead it and bake it. Well, maybe they're not growing or picking it, but they do have huge 50# buckets full of various kinds of wheat that they grind in a machine that is guaranteed to shatter your ear drums if you get too close. It will also make the most incredible bread you have ever tasted in all your born days.

I am not yet in that place in my life where I am grinding my own. As a matter of fact, I am just starting to get over the intimidation factor of yeast and realizing that making your own pizza isn't a big deal. Making bread isn't either, especially if your indentured servant (the Automatic Bread Machine) is doing all the work.

I don't want you to spend your cooking years being intimidated by yeast like I was. Use your indentured servant and enjoy what wonderful things yeast can make. Here are some quick pointers that will help you understand this mysterious substance a little better:

• Yeast doesn't like too hot or too cold of water. Lukewarm—the temp should be right around 100 to 115 degrees—less hot if you're using a bread machine.

• Not all yeasts are created equal. I have really enjoyed using the bulk yeast I bought from the health food store and my friend Vickilynn Haycraft, who in my opinion, knows her stuff when it comes to all things related to breadmaking, thinks SAF brand is the best around.

• Any questions about the quality of your yeast will come out if you "proof" it. The proof is in the pudding, as they say. Dissolve the yeast in about ¼ cup warm water and let it stand about 5 minutes. Add a little honey (about a teaspoon) and some flour (about 2 tablespoons) and within 10 minutes you should see activity—it will foam and expand, otherwise it's dead and you need some fresh stuff.

• While yeast is fed by the honey and grows in the flour, kneading is what causes the gluten in the wheat to develop and what makes the dough look sort of stringy and elastic in texture. If you're making Presto Pretzels *page 161*, you can teach this to your child. If you're using your indentured servant on the "dough" setting, at least you know what's going on in there. If you're making bread by hand, you're a better woman than I am.

• I mentioned gluten in the glossary, but I'll mention it again. Buying a package of this stuff from the health food store will save your bread from being an adobe brick and your pizza from being tough and overly chewy. It's inexpensive and lasts forever. I keep mine in the fridge. Add about a tablespoon of this per cup or so of flour.

Now see? That wasn't so bad, was it?

Just the Flax Ma'am Muffins

I can almost hear Joe Friday saying this…"Just the flax, Ma'am. We just need the flax."
Now listen up here, the flax in this recipe is only for the fiber. By baking these, the EFA' bake right out. Don't eat
the dough raw, though. Try the Crockpot Cereal with raw flax for the EFA benefits. Makes 36 muffins

3 cups kamut flour
1 ½ cups flax seeds, ground
1 ½ cups oat bran
4 teaspoons baking powder
2 teaspoons baking soda
2 teaspoons sea salt
2 teaspoons cinnamon
1 teaspoon nutmeg
1 ½ cups buttermilk
¼ cup safflower oil
1 ½ cups honey
4 eggs, beaten
4 teaspoons vanilla
4 cups carrots, shredded (or zucchini)
4 apples, peeled and chopped
½ cup each raisins or/and nuts, very op-
tional—we never use 'em

Preheat oven to 350 degrees. Prepare muffin pan by greasing or lining with paper cupcake liners.

In a large bowl, toss together the dry ingredients (first 8 ingredients) and make a well in the middle.

In another bowl, mix together the buttermilk, honey, eggs and vanilla. Add to the dry ingredients and mix till incorporated. Add carrot (or zucchini) and apple and nuts and/or raisins, if you choose to use them.

Fill muffin cups 2/3 full and bake for 18-20 minutes, but like I always say, CHECK THEM! Ovens can do funny things, you never know sometimes…Cool in the pan for 5 minutes, then pop from the pan and transfer to a wire rack to finish cooling.

PER SERVING: 189 CALORIES (KCAL); 5G TOTAL FAT; (21% CALORIES FROM FAT); 5G PROTEIN; 35G CARBOHYDRATE; 21MG CHOLESTEROL; 253MG SODIUM

COOKING NOTES: If you are going to go to all the trouble of making these, you might as well make mass quantities and freeze. They aren't hard to make, or even that time consuming—there's just a lot of ingredients. Well worth the effort though.

Mayberry Blueberry Muffins

So Aunt Bea would use sugar...she also wore a girdle and nylons baking...case closed.

12 muffins

1 cup kamut flour
¾ cup whole wheat pastry flour
¾ cup organic sucanat
4 teaspoons baking powder
2 teaspoons lemon juice
¾ cup buttermilk, or add 1 teaspoon
   vinegar to milk to make it sour
1 teaspoon vanilla extract
¼ cup safflower oil
1 cup blueberries, frozen or fresh

Preheat oven to 400 degrees. Prepare muffin tin by greasing or lining with paper cupcake liners.

In a large bowl, mix together dry ingredients, and make a well in the center. In a separate bowl, mix wet ingredients well and add to dry ingredients. Mix till combined.

Gently fold in the berries

Spoon batter into prepared muffin tin, filling each cup ¾ full.

Bake for 18-20 minutes. Cool for 5 minutes in muffin tin, then remove individual muffins and place on a wire rack to cool.

PER SERVING: 173 CALORIES (KCAL); 5G TOTAL FAT; (24% CALORIES FROM FAT); 3G PROTEIN; 32G CARBOHYDRATE; 1MG CHOLESTEROL, 179MG SODIUM

"I loved these! My five-year-old son could easily qualify as the world's pickiest eater. With normal blueberry muffins he picks out the blueberries and leaves behind the muffins. He ate these muffins! I couldn't believe it! Delicious!"—Robin Schneider

Mega Manic Muffin Mix

If muffins aren't just the most wonderful things for breakfast...I just LOVE the versatility and cheapness of it all! This mix makes 'em hearty and full of fiber.

Yield: 120 Muffins

10 cups whole wheat pastry flour

5 cups kamut flour

5 cups sucanat

2 cups buttermilk, dried

2 cups oats, pulverized in a food processor

6 tablespoons baking powder

2 tablespoons baking soda

2 tablespoons sea salt

Mix all ingredients well and keep in a sealed container.

To make a basic muffin, use 5 ½ cup of muffin mix and add 2 eggs, 2 egg whites, 3 tsp. vanilla, 2 cups water, ½ cup safflower oil, to make a batch of 24 muffins. All varieties can be baked in prepared tins, 18-20 minutes in a pre-heated 400 degree oven.

PER SERVING: 76 CALORIES (KCAL); TRACE TOTAL FAT; (2% CALORIES FROM FAT); 2G PROTEIN; 18G CARBOHYDRATE; 1MG CHOLESTEROL; 240MG SODIUM

VARIATIONS: This is only the base of your muffin recipe. There are 800 variations on this theme, made possible by you, the chef, the cook, the muffin maker extraordinaire.

One or two ideas are here just to launch you into a creative frenzy, causing you to create mega-muffins with flair. Try these variations and see if you can't think up a few of your own.

Apple Pie Muffins

2 ½ cups grated apple

1 teaspoon cinnamon

½ teaspoon nutmeg

Gingerbread-style Muffins

¼ cup blackstrap molasses

2 tablespoons ground ginger

Jam Muffins

Add a teaspoon of fruit juice sweetened conserve to the middle, by pouring half your muffin mix, plopping a blob of conserve and filling with a little more mix.

Maple Pecan Muffins

6 tablespoons of pure maple syrup

Use only 1 ½ cups of water instead

1 cup of chopped pecans.

"The muffin mix was tremendous. We made chunky fruity muffins for our first batch using an assortment of dried fruits I had just purchased—dried cherries, cranberries, dates, blueberries, raisins, apples, papaya and cantaloupe (my daughter added that one.) My older kids didn't want to be out done, so they made pizza muffins. They used the basic muffin mix, added cheese to the batter and filled the muffin tins half full. They added pizza sauce and more cheese, topped with more batter and baked until brown. You can add just about anything to this mild tasting mix and have it turn out wonderfully." —Kathy Beaver

Over-the-Top Muffin Toppers

Love that streusel stuff on the top of muffins? Who doesn't!

1 batch

1 cup oats
½ cup oat bran
½ cup whole wheat pastry flour
½ cup sucanat
2 teaspoons cinnamon
½ cup unsalted butter, very cold, sliced 1"
    thick

In a food processor, place all dry ingredients, pulse to mix.

Lay butter slices out all over the top of the mixture. Pulse till it looks chunky, like granola.

Use on your muffin recipe and save any leftovers in a freezer bag and freeze.

PER RECIPE: 736 CALORIES (KCAL); 14G TOTAL FAT; (15% CALORIES FROM FAT); 35G PROTEIN, 138G CARBOHYDRATE; 0MG CHOLESTEROL; 6MG SODIUM

Peach Spiced French Toast Strata

This will knock everyone's socks off and have them begging for the recipe. Don't give in. Keep this one to yourself. Everyone needs a secret weapon.

Serves 12

1 loaf wheat bread

8 eggs

3 cups milk, 1% low-fat

1 teaspoon nutmeg

1 tablespoon vanilla

3 cups sliced peaches, frozen, fresh or canned is fine

1 cup organic sucanat

2 tablespoons unsalted butter

Preheat oven to 350 degrees. Grease a 13 x 9 inch pan. Chop up bread and fit on the bottom of baking pan.

In a bowl, beat remaining ingredients but only half the sucanat and no peaches. Pour over the top of the bread and let sit for a while. (Stratas traditionally sit overnight in your fridge, but I don't like it that way.) Give your strata at least an hour to soak. In the meantime, do your nails, floss your teeth or call an old friend. Okay, now that you're back, top the strata with the peaches, sprinkle with remaining sucanat and dot with butter.

Bake for about an hour, although, if you're smart you'll watch it. Nothing worse than overcooked strata. Don't ask me how I know that.

PER SERVING: 188 CALORIES (KCAL); 6G TOTAL FAT; (26% CALORIES FROM FAT); 6G PROTEIN; 29G CARBOHYDRATE; 132MG CHOLESTEROL; 79MG SODIUM

"I wasn't so sure about a peach strata, but I gave it a whirl. To my surprise and delight, we loved it! Everyone gave it a '10' rating. The only problem is, we can't decide if we like it better fresh from the oven all light and airy, or cooled and denser-textured, or whether we should have it for breakfast, brunch, afternoon snack or dessert. So, I'll let you decide and I'll go put my feet up and enjoy a cup of tea and a hunk of this great peach strata! By the way, this reheats beautifully in the oven, uncovered in a casserole dish at 350°F for about 20 minutes depending on how many pieces you reheat." —Vickilynn Haycraft.

Pumpkin Mumpkins

This recipe screams Autumn, but don't just eat them then. This is a muffin to be enjoyed anytime of year.
Makes 18 muffins

2 ½ cups kamut flour
1 cup organic sucanat
1 tablespoon pumpkin pie spice
1 teaspoon baking soda
¼ teaspoon sea salt
1 cup pumpkin, canned
¼ cup safflower oil
2 cups apple, chopped.
2 eggs

Preheat oven to 350 degrees. Prepare muffin tin by greasing or lining with cupcake papers.

In a large bowl, combine dry ingredients. Make a well in the middle.

In a smaller bowl, mix well wet ingredients.

Add wet to dry, mixing well to incorporate.

Spoon batter into muffin cups ¾ full. Bake for 25-30 minutes, checking ever so often.

Remove from oven and cool in tin for 5 minutes. Remove from pan and finish cooling on a rack.

PER SERVING: 200 CALORIES (KCAL); 4G TOTAL FAT; (17% CALORIES FROM FAT); 5G PROTEIN; 40G CARBOHYDRATE; 21MG CHOLESTEROL; 103MG SODIUM

"Moist and sweet with a very nice pumpkin spice flavor—
my kids are begging me to make these again today." —Sue LeMay

Smoothie Patrol

Here are some general guidelines for making awesome smoothies. My rule of thumb is to use what I have on hand. Of course, I always have lots on hand!

Serves 1

2 ounces tofu, I buy the silkened tofu
1 banana, frozen
¼ cup berries, frozen
1 scoop protein powder
1 teaspoon vanilla extract
1/3 cup orange juice

Put everything in a blender and LET HER RIP!

COOKING NOTES: For the berries option, you could use peaches, some more banana whatever. Smoothies are pretty forgiving—the only necessary component is frozen fruit to make it shake-like. If you have a muffin and smoothie for breakfast, you're set to go till lunch.

PER SERVING: 216 CALORIES (KCAL); 4G TOTAL FAT; (14% CALORIES FROM FAT); 7G PROTEIN; 41G CARBOHYDRATE; 2MG CHOLESTEROL; 12MG SODIUM

Smoothie Stuff

There are smoothie recipes, and I even gave you one, but from where I sit, a mom (a busy mom, just like a lot of you) I don't have the time to measure all this stuff out. So, read these guidelines and develop your own smoothies. They just take a second to whip up and they make a great drink to go—like on the way to soccer practice, for example.

Here are some quick guidelines:

First, remember everything goes in a blender. Make sure you don't float the protein powder on top or it won't blend. Keep in my mind your blender's capacity—my blender tops out at two big smoothies.

Here are some suggestions for ingredients:

1 Something sweet. You know how your bananas get all icky with fruit flies because they're past their prime? Don't toss them! Freeze them, just as they are. (you could go to the trouble of peeling and sticking them in a bag, but why bother?) After they freeze, they'll turn black, just on the outside, though. Use a paring knife like you're peeling the skin off a cucumber and put the frozen banana in the blender—about a half per person.

2 Something for flavor. I sometimes use a teaspoon of frozen orange juice concentrate, per person. That works. Sometimes frozen strawberries, raspberries—whatever.

3 Something for liquid. I use soy milk, because my daughter is allergic to dairy. You could use regular milk, juice, yogurt even, with some water.

4 Something for extra protein. I use a scoop per person of protein powder. I am currently using GNC brand, but just look on the label of any health food store protein powders. You want high protein, low carbs (you already have all the carbs you need in the fruit) and NO aspartame—ick.

Gentlemen, (and ladies) Start Your Engines! (turn on the blender). You should have a delicious smoothie emerging shortly. Get a spoon and taste it. If you followed these insipid directions, it should be a tasty orange or berry/banana smoothie. You could also throw a little vanilla extract in—that's a nice touch. In any case, together with a muffin, you have one great breakfast.

Stuffed French Toast

Definitely week-end food, but what a treat!
Serves 8

4 ounces low-fat cream cheese
2 tablespoons orange juice
1 tablespoon orange zest
4 eggs
1 cup skim milk
1/8 cup organic sucanat
1/8 teaspoon nutmeg
½ teaspoon cinnamon
8 slices whole wheat bread
1 teaspoon vanilla extract
2 teaspoons unsalted butter
½ cup apricot spreadable fruit
2 tablespoons honey

In a bowl, place cream cheese, orange juice and orange zest. Beat till smooth.

In another bowl, beat eggs, milk, vanilla, sucanat and spices.

Heat non-stick pan and swirl a little butter around for the French toast to cook in. Cut the whole grain bread in half and soak in custard mixture.

Cook evenly and set in a 200 degree oven to keep warm. Make apricot honey topping by combining apricot conserve and honey and warming till thinned.

On each plate, take the ½ piece of French Toast and top with an ounce of cream cheese mixture. Top with another ½ piece of French Toast and drizzle with apricot honey topping.

PER SERVING: 220 CALORIES (KCAL); 7G TOTAL FAT; (27% CALORIES FROM FAT); 8G PROTEIN; 32G CARBOHYDRATE; 105MG CHOLESTEROL; 275MG SODIUM

"My kids loved this, even my son who does not like French Toast—quite tasty!" Christina Fredricks

Yummy Yogurt Bowl

Don't underestimate the value of yogurt, but don't buy the yucky, commercial artificially colored stuff either. If you can't make your own, get plain. Here's how to make it right.

Serves 4

2 cups nonfat yogurt
1 cup frozen blueberries, or any berry.
1 banana, sliced
1 cup granola—you could also use Grape
**   Nuts cereal. In any case, use low-fat.**
½ cup raisin
2 tablespoons honey

In a large mixing bowl, mix together all ingredients. Don't thaw blueberries—they are wonderful to eat crunchy and frozen like that. Divvy up and serve.

PER SERVING: 345 CALORIES (KCAL); 6G TOTAL FAT; (21% CALORIES FROM FAT); 11G PROTEIN; 60G CARBOHYDRATE; 2MG CHOLESTEROL; 93MG SODIUM

"Creamy, fruity and super protein source. My nine-year-old daughter, Clancy, loved it!" —Dana O'Sullivan

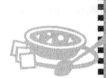

Soup and Salad Bar

I am not one of those that believes soup should be served for a first course. First courses are for people who have butlers. The soups and salads in this section are good and hearty enough for a main course. So don't skip this section in search of more substantial food. Enjoy these soups and salads—they're some of my family's favorites.

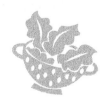

Cheesy Broccoli Soup

*Describing anything but this soup as cheesy, most certainly would be
insulting. Check this soup out—kids LOVE it!*
Serves 4 (or more)

2 onions, chopped
**3 cups broccoli, chopped, stems and all
    (fresh or frozen)**
3 cloves garlic, crushed
1 tablespoon olive oil
**1 quart chicken broth, canned or home-
    made**
1 cup cheddar cheese, low-fat, shredded
1 cup milk, skim

In a large soup pot, sauté onions and garlic till wilted.
Add chopped broccoli and continue cooking.

Pour broth over the top and cook till broccoli is
very tender, about ½ hour.

In batches, process soup through a food processor or
blender till almost smooth. Some chunks are nice.

Add milk and let continue cooking another 20 minutes, but be careful not to let boil or the soup will
separate.

When nice and thick, remove from heat and serve
in individual bowls. Top each bowl with ¼ cup cheddar cheese and serve with a great, big salad and whole
grain bread. Great dinner!

PER SERVING: 178 CALORIES (KCAL); 7G TOTAL FAT; (35% CALORIES
FROM FAT); 16G PROTEIN; 13G CARBOHYDRATE; 7MG CHOLESTEROL;
984MG SODIUM

*"This is a great recipe! My three daughters all liked it. It did sneak up to boiling on me, after the milk was in the soup, but I
guess it didn't get too hot too long, because it didn't separate."*—Bonnie Musselwhite

Crock-potato Cheese Soup

This is a recipe my ten year old daughter makes for us. It's an easy, delicious recipe that will fill you up.

Serves 6

2 pounds potatoes, peeled and cubed
1 onion, chopped
5 cups chicken broth or vegetable broth
salt and pepper to taste
1 cup milk, 1% low-fat, or use soy milk
1 cup cheddar cheese, low-fat, shredded

Cook the first three ingredients, with the salt and pepper in a crockpot for 3 hours on high (or until done).

Process half the potato mixture in a food processor, pour into a pot and add remaining crock potted potato mixture. Stir well and heat, adding milk. When the soup begins to simmer, turn down the heat. If it boils too hard, the soup will separate. Correct the seasoning. Lest you think I add thyme, garlic powder and salt and pepper to every soup I make, I have omitted it here. Although feel free to add it yourself.

Ladle up a good-sized portion and top with some cheddar cheese. Serve.

PER SERVING: 176 CALORIES (KCAL); 2G TOTAL FAT; (9% CALORIES FROM FAT); 9G PROTEIN; 31G CARBOHYDRATE; 6MG CHOLESTEROL; 145MG SODIUM

"A simple and delicious soup, my picky 8 year old asked for seconds, and even the baby said 'mmmmm!' This would be a good no-fuss for anyone. Put ingredients in crockpot at breakfast...ready to eat at lunch!"
—Marya Mesa

"The potato cheese soup smelled so good cooking I loved the taste — the taste is great like 'grandma-great taters' that you could never figure out what her secret ingredient was. This is perfect for those busy cold days."—Lori Sparks

Lentil Soup

More like a stew, this soup is very satisfying. Lentil soup is something I absolutely crave in the middle of winter. A hot bowl of soup, homemade bread and a tossed green salad. A perfect dinner.

Serves 8

1 pound lentils, rinsed, drained and picked over

2 onions , chopped

2 carrots, chopped

5 cups chicken broth

1 teaspoon thyme

**1 teaspoon garlic powder,
   or use 1 clove fresh garlic**

1 can diced tomato

salt and pepper to taste

In a soup pot, add a little oil and sauté vegetables. Add remaining ingredients and simmer for an hour.

OR throw everything together in a crockpot, turn on low and serve it up nine hours later. If you like a thicker, creamier-type soup and less bumps, feel free to puree a part of the soup in the blender. I don't, but some prefer it this way.

PER SERVING: 229 CALORIES (KCAL); 2G TOTAL FAT; (5% CALORIES FROM FAT); 19G PROTEIN; 36G CARBOHYDRATE; 0MG CHOLESTEROL; 491MG SODIUM

"I made this tasty recipe according to the crockpot instructions, making it an easy meal with just a few things to round it out. It smelled great cooking all day. We thought it was more like saucy lentils and Tim said the taste was 'soothing' and 'goes down easy'. He gave it a '10'. I would smash up the lentils a bit, but other than that we really liked it. This would be great for a busy day meal. Leftovers were just as good for lunch and this freezes well too!"

—Vickilynn Haycraft

Pistou Vegetable Soup

I fell in love with this soup eons ago and crafted this version of it to fit my family.
Serves 12

1 pound dried white beans, cooked (you can use any white beans you have on hand)
1 tablespoon olive oil
2 onions, chopped
4 cloves garlic
3 carrots, chopped
1 celery rib, chopped
4 potatoes, diced
1-28 ounces can of whole tomatoes, diced
¼ head cabbage, shredded
8 leaves kale, shredded
6 cups chicken broth, canned or homemade

1 teaspoon thyme
salt and pepper to taste
Pesto (see page 86)

Puree half the beans in your food processor and set aside.

In a large pot, heat olive oil and sauté onion and garlic for about two minutes or till translucent. Add carrot, celery and potato and sauté another 2 minutes.

Add tomatoes and their liquid, beans, bean puree, and seasoning. Let simmer 5 minutes. Add chicken broth to the mixture (sooner if it seems to be drying out) .

Add cabbage and kale, correct the seasoning and serve with a dollop of pesto on the top.

PER SERVING: 114 CALORIES (KCAL); 2G TOTAL FAT; (18% CALORIES FROM FAT); 6G PROTEIN; 19G CARBOHYDRATE; 0MG CHOLESTEROL; 419MG SODIUM

"My family loved this hearty soup and didn't even know they liked kale!
Just add a crisp green salad and a good loaf of bread for a great vegetarian meal."
—Dana O'Sullivan

Pesto

Pesto packs a punch in the flavor department, almost like nothing else. It's high in fat, though, so a little goes a long way. Use judiciously.

Serves 24

4 cloves garlic

4 ounces Romano cheese, cut in 1" pieces

¾ cup pine nuts (pignolia)

2 cups basil leaves

¾ cup olive oil

salt and pepper to taste

In a food processor, place the first 3 ingredients and let her rip.

Next, add basil and pulse till combined and chopped. Add olive oil in a slow stream with machine running.

Scrape out of the bowl and use or store in ice cube trays in the freezer till molded. Then pull your pesto cubes out and stack them in freezer bags and throw them back in the freezer.

PER SERVING: 103 CALORIES (KCAL); 10G TOTAL FAT; (87% CALORIES FROM FAT); 3G PROTEIN; 1G CARBOHYDRATE; 5MG CHOLESTEROL; 38MG SODIUM

Chinese Cole Slaw with Ginger Chicken

Forgive me if this is redundant having TWO recipes for Chinese Cole Slaw in the same book, but it's great stuff. Fairly versatile and keeps better than a tossed green salad, right?

Serves 6

16 ounces cabbage, shredded
3 green onions, chopped
3 teaspoons ginger, grated
2 cloves garlic, pressed
1 tablespoon soy sauce, low sodium
1 tablespoon sesame oil
2 tablespoons rice wine vinegar
1 tablespoon lime juice
¼ cup mayonnaise, low-fat

Place cabbage and green onion in a large bowl.

In another bowl, whisk together remaining ingredients and pour over cabbage mixture.

Toss, cover and refrigerate, allowing flavors to meld for at least an hour. Then serve with sliced, chilled ginger chicken. *(see page 88)*

PER SERVING: 94 CALORIES (KCAL); 7G TOTAL FAT; (62% CALORIES FROM FAT); 2G PROTEIN, 8G CARBOHYDRATE; 0MG CHOLESTEROL; 148MG SODIUM

"Easy to prepare and very quick to eat. A refreshing change from the Deli style coleslaw that is dripping with mayonnaise. With a family that enjoys flavorful and spicy foods. I like it if they are easy to prepare."—Carol Reynolds.

Ginger Chicken

Very easy to make and quick recipe to boot.
Use with one of the Chinese Cole Slaw recipes for an easy, summer meal.
Serves 4

4 boneless, skinless chicken breasts
4 teaspoons soy sauce or Tamari—use low
   salt if available
1 tablespoon ginger, fresh is great, but if
   you don't have it, powdered works fine
2 cloves garlic, pressed
¼ cup rice wine vinegar

Put all ingredients in a big plastic bag and mush it around periodically in the fridge. Let marinate a couple of hours, at least.

Fire up the barby! Cook when the coals are red hot or preheat oven to 350 degrees. Dump the whole bag (not the bag though) into a baking dish and cook your chicken till done, about 20 minutes or so depending on size and thickness.

Note: Very gingery. If you don't like too much ginger, feel free to decrease the ginger.

PER SERVING: 291 CALORIES (KCAL); 6G TOTAL FAT; (19% CALORIES FROM FAT); 53G PROTEIN; 3G CARBOHYDRATE; 144MG CHOLESTEROL; 461MG SODIUM

"Ginger Chicken is a winner and was quickly gone, with looks of 'is there more?'—Carol Reynolds

Mexican Chicken Salad

More Fast Food—can't get any easier than this!
Serves 4

1 bag salad—like organic baby greens or whatever you like

8 ounces chicken or taco meat , use left-overs

½ can black beans, drained

1 tomato, diced

½ bunch cilantro, chopped, optional

6 ounces low-fat cheddar cheese, grated

½ cup salsa

low-fat or nonfat sour cream

2 green onions, minced

4 tablespoons vinaigrette

In a large mixing bowl, toss all ingredients but the sour cream, cheese and sour cream. Serve salad on to 4 plates.

Evenly distribute chicken on the salad plates. Garnish with sour cream and cilantro and cheese.

PER SERVING: 245 CALORIES (KCAL); 11G TOTAL FAT; (40% CALORIES FROM FAT); 16G PROTEIN; 20G CARBOHYDRATE; 9MG CHOLESTEROL; 406MG SODIUM

"We all loved the Mexican Chicken Salad. It was a real hit! We had company the night I served it and it went over really well. It was so quick to prepare, but looked and tasted like a restaurant style entree (Especially because I served it on baby greens)." —Lisa Young

Salad Nicoise

A French cafe classic with a few distinct differences.
Serves 6

1 head romaine lettuce, washed and patted dry

2 tomato, diced

2 eggs, hard-boiled, diced

1 can tuna in water, well drained

1 pound green beans, steamed

1 red onion, diced fine

10 new potatoes, cooked and quartered

Nicoise olives, optional

½ cup vinaigrette, homemade (see page 94) or bottled

In a large bowl, place all ingredients except lettuce and toss well. Set aside and let sit for 10 minutes while you prepare the lettuce.

Tear lettuce into bowl on top of your marinating mixture and toss well. Serve.

PER SERVING: 368 CALORIES (KCAL); 13G TOTAL FAT; (30% CALORIES FROM FAT); 17G PROTEIN; 49G CARBOHYDRATE; 78MG CHOLESTEROL; 139MG SODIUM

Tabbouleh

I made this about every other day when I went through my vegetarian stage in the 80's. This is wonderful!
Serves 8

1 cup bulgur wheat
1 cup water, boiling
2 tomatoes, chopped
2 green onions, chopped
½ cup parsley, chopped fine
¼ cup mint, chopped fine
¼ cup lemon juice
1/8 cup olive oil
1 clove garlic, pressed

In a bowl, stir bulgur wheat and boiling water together and let sit while you chop.

In another bowl, mix lemon juice, olive oil and garlic to make dressing. After everything is chopped, add it to the bowl and toss together.

Drizzle dressing over the top and toss again. Refrigerate till cool, then serve.

COOKING NOTES: If you want to use this as a main course, slice up some chicken and put it in the salad. Will serve 4 generously as a main dish.

PER SERVING: 102 CALORIES (KCAL); 4G TOTAL FAT; (30% CALORIES FROM FAT); 3G PROTEIN; 16G CARBOHYDRATE; 0MG CHOLESTEROL; 10MG SODIUM

Ode to Garlic

Garlic, garlic, garlic fair—When I eat you, people stare
Garlic, garlic, bulb odiferous—I like you much on vegetables cruciferous.

Garlic does tend to be somewhat, um, aromatic, doesn't it? But what an aroma it is! And the best news? Not only does it do wondrously, flavorful things in the kitchen, it is so incredibly good for you, too. Garlic made the rounds a couple of years back, as the new darling of the traditional medical community, if you remember. I snickered at the time (okay—I smirked), having known this for quite awhile, as I give garlic due credit in helping my daughter get over chronic ear infections when the doctors couldn't.

For the sake of review for the initiated or if this is new news for the newbies, let's take a look at some of garlic's redeeming qualities. Garlic's potent ingredient is called allicin. Allicin is the antifungal, antibiotic-like property of garlic that helps heal you from the inside out, by aiding and stimulating the immune system. Garlic also helps lower cholesterol levels, aids in digestion and lowers blood pressure.

During mosquito season here in North Carolina, I double up on my garlic supplement to avoid becoming a human buffet for those bloodthirsty pests. Yep, it's true! Garlic keeps away little, flying vampires. It's supposed to work on animals too, although I cannot figure that one out considering the fact that dogs and cats pant when hot, and don't sweat. Maybe someone can clue me in on that.

People who are prone to cold sores, athlete's foot and any kind of fungal infection, would do well to include a garlic supplement in their diet, as well as cooking with garlic. The delicate allicin is mostly killed off by cooking though, so you need to eat your garlic raw. Caesar salads are great for that and what could be better than a main course salad during warm summer months? I have a wonderful recipe, Very Garlic-y Chicken Caesar Salad (*page 93*) that will not only help you get more raw garlic in your diet, but give you an enjoyable way to do it.

Just remember to make this a family affair. That way, no one will be offended by your garlic-y "presence".

Very Garlic-y Chicken Caesar Salad

Garlic lovers unite! Here is your salad. You'll have to go into hiding after you eat it though, the garlic is rather pungent.

Serves 4

12 ounces chicken breast without skin, grilled or use leftovers
1 head romaine lettuce, chopped
½ cup croutons
2 cloves garlic, pressed
2 teaspoons lemon juice
½ teaspoon Dijon mustard
2 ounces anchovy fillet
1/8 cup Romano cheese
2 tablespoons red wine vinegar
¼ cup olive oil
1 teaspoon Worcestershire sauce

Make croutons first by chopping up stale bread, brushing with olive oil and sprinkling with a little garlic powder. Toast in 350 degree oven till brown—probably no more than 10 minutes. Check them often, though!

Wash romaine and chop into bite-sized pieces. Normally, you only want to tear lettuce, but if you are going to be using it right away, chop away and save yourself some time.

In a bowl, combine oil, vinegar, Worcestershire, salt and pepper to taste, garlic, lemon juice, anchovies and mustard. Or use the food processor (that's what I do).

In a large bowl, toss lettuce and dressing and half the cheese together along with your croutons. Serve on individual plates and top with chicken and remaining cheese.

PER SERVING: 286 CALORIES (KCAL); 13G TOTAL FAT; (53% CALORIES FROM FAT); 25G PROTEIN; 9G CARBOHYDRATE; 55MG CHOLESTEROL; 669MG SODIUM

Vinaigrette

This is a classic with a few healthy updates. Makes about 2/3 cup.

1 tablespoon Dijon mustard
4 tablespoons balsamic vinegar
1 teaspoon honey
½ teaspoon sea salt
½ cup olive oil
fresh ground pepper

In a bowl, plop all ingredients, except olive oil. Using a wire whisk, mix all ingredients well.

Keep whisking and add olive oil in a steady stream. That's all there is to it. Lasts approximately two weeks when stored in refrigerator.

COOKING NOTES: *Variations on a Theme*—You can add a clove of pressed garlic to make a garlic vinaigrette, snip fresh herbs in it or even change out the vinegar for a different flavor. For an Asian flavor, try changing out the balsamic for rice wine vinegar and use ½ olive oil and 2 tablespoons of sesame oil.

PER RECIPE: 997 CALORIES (KCAL); 109G TOTAL FAT; (95% CALORIES FROM FAT); 1G PROTEIN; 11G CARBOHYDRATE; 0MG CHOLESTEROL; 1129MG SODIUM

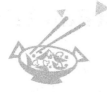

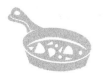

Life in the Fast Food Lane

Lest you think I've totally lost it, let me give you an important preamble to this cooking section. This is about making your own fast food, not an invitation to a BK triple cheeseburger. All the recipes in this section were designed for those nights when it's just got to be quick and every second counts.

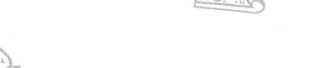

Avocado Yumwich

Avocados have been given the nutritional shaft over their fat content. That's good fat, especially for kids. Most kids love avocado. Here's a great recipe, perfect for lunch.

Serves 1

2 slices whole wheat bread, any whole grain bread will do
¼ avocado
½ ounce low-fat cream cheese
1 slice tomato

Put together and eat. How's that for cinchy instructions? For gooooood eatin', slice onions up and sauté till brown. When they're still working on their tans, add a little barbeque sauce and add that to your yumwich. Eat with wild abandon.

PER SERVING: 277 CALORIES (KCAL); 13G TOTAL FAT; (39% CALORIES FROM FAT); 9G PROTEIN; 36G CARBOHYDRATE; 8MG CHOLESTEROL; 410MG SODIUM

"My husband needed something he could eat in the minivan this evening, so my daughter Michelle fixed him this sandwich. He says, 'It's a light, delicious vegetarian sandwich— the Yumwich keeps 'em asking for more!'" —Lee Ann Roberts

Snack Attack

Let's be reasonable. You make dinner, you pack lunches, you grocery shop, chop, cook and slave over a hot stove. Why on earth should anyone have to "make" snacks? There ought to be a law...

I haven't heard of any laws recently, but I do know a good snack when I see one. Here's a list of quick and easy snacks.

• **Cottage cheese**—don't overlook this great food. Of course, if milk allergies are a problem, do overlook it. Topped with a little honey or sliced fruit, it's a great snack.

• **Yogurt.** I did include a recipe of sorts for a yogurt bowl. The only reason was so you wouldn't forget about this highly nutritious food.

• **Veggie patrol.** Unless you have little kids, let your big kid wash and peel his own carrot. They like doing this and it's a great, good for you snack. There are lots of veggies in the produce department that you can buy already ready to go. The baby carrots are a good example. Good time to whip out the dips.

• **Fruit.** Keep an accessible basket or bowl of fruit on your kitchen table or counter. That's a good place for kids to grab a snack. Ours is always heavily loaded with bananas and apples. Those two fruits are pretty much standard issue year 'round, but I'll throw something seasonal in there when it's on sale, too.

• **Cheese cubes.** Get out those sticks! Perfect food for On-A-Stick. Use low-fat cheeses, though. Same flavor and nutrients, less fat.

• **Slice of whole grain bread** with a smear of peanut or almond butter. That'll hold 'em till dinner time.

• Banana sliced down the middle with peanut butter in it. Encourage kids to eat this mess outside.

• **Banana frozen** and (you guessed it) On-A-Stick.

• **Dried fruit**—maybe just a handful of raisins. My kids like prunes stuck on all five fingers—I don't mind if they're outside and I don't have to watch.

• **A muffin from the freezer.** If you're smart, you've doubled and tripled the recipes in this book and have a bounty in your freezer.

• **Popcorn** don't even *think* about the microwaveable kind—very unhealthy. Use a hot air popper and go for it.

• **Retro Granola bars**, Puffy Cereal bars, I do have a few recipes in this book. Mind you, I hope you've made these for lunch boxes, a special event or even a child training cooking "class" at home. Don't you be knocking yourself out trying to cook all day long, morning, noon and night.

• **Cool Fruits** makes some terrific, healthy snacks of all kinds—my favorite was the pumpcorn—pumpkin seeds with chili flavoring. They have a bunch of stuff—all easy to order over the internet. Their site is www.coolfruits.com.

• Another place to nab some good snacks is **Village Organics**. They have all the usual stuff you'll find in a well-stocked health food store, without the hassle of having to go in. You can order from their secured server on the internet, www.villageorganics.com . Even their packing material is environmentally friendly!

• **Skeet and Ikes** have done wondrous things to soybeans. After roasting soybeans, they are flavored with honey dijon mustard, yogurt and green onion, BBQ, or just plain sea salt. Interesting, crunchy snacks. Check them out at: www.skeetike.com

• **Water.** If you gave your child a snack and he is still complaining about being hungry, and he's eaten enough to satisfy him, don't give him anything else. He's probably thirsty. One of the places where we can get seriously confused is not being able to discern hunger from thirst. Let him have water first.

Basic Beans

To make recipe ready beans and to cut down on the cans, try this easy method for getting beans cooked. It's much less expensive to use dried beans. Do this with a bunch of beans and freeze when done.

Serves 8

1 pound dried beans, rinsed and drained, picked clean
5 cups water, boiled

Put clean beans in your crockpot, bring a kettle to boil and pour over the top. Cook for 3 to 4 hours on high, depending on the size of the bean or cook on low 5 to 7 hours.

When cooked, drain and rinse well in a colander. Use for recipe or store in bags in the freezer, labeled and dated, of course.

PER SERVING: 190 CALORIES (KCAL); 1G TOTAL FAT; (3% CALORIES FROM FAT); 13G PROTEIN; 34G CARBOHYDRATE; 0MG CHOLESTEROL; 12MG SODIUM

Cowboy Beans

My kids like these with cornbread and a bottle of barbeque sauce right on the table.
Serves 8

1 pound pinto beans, rinsed, drained and picked over

5 cups water, boiled

2 onions, chopped

1 cup barbeque sauce, Hain makes a good one

2 squirts ketchup

1 carrot, grated

2 squirts mustard

salt and pepper to taste

In a crockpot, mix beans, water and onion. Cook on high for 3-4 hours. Then cook on low for 7 hours or so.

Drain beans and add the barbeque sauce and ketchup and mustard squirts. Salt and pepper to taste. Mix it up and serve it in bowls with plenty of cornbread and honey butter. A huge green salad makes the meal. Or serve greens on the side with rice wine vinegar. All you need is a campfire and your sleeve as a napkin.

PER SERVING: 212 CALORIES (KCAL); 1G TOTAL FAT; (3% CALORIES FROM FAT); 12G PROTEIN; 40G CARBOHYDRATE; 0MG CHOLESTEROL; 70MG SODIUM

"Here it is, almost the end of the month and there are more healthy meals to make before payday. The fresh vegetables are history, the month's beef purchases are just a memory and these days supper is procured by gathering what's available on the homestead or doing some 'pantry diving'. So, I says to Leanne, I says, 'sure, I'll test a recipe IF it has ingredients that are whole grains, fresh eggs or goat milk, or foods that are canned, frozen or dried.' This recipe works wonderfully and was a hit! It was very filling and satisfying served with side dishes. Joshua gave it an 8.5."—Vickilynn Haycraft

Crunchy Honey Mustard Chicken Fingers

Totally 100% kid food. Parents can eat these too, but you'll probably need to make more!

Serves 4

1 pound chicken breasts, no skin, no bone
¼ cup honey , warmed
¼ cup Dijon mustard
1 cup corn flakes, crushed

Preheat oven to 425 degrees. Lightly grease a cookie sheet.

In a small bowl, mix mustard and warm honey together well. Put crushed corn flakes in a separate bowl.

Slice chicken into ¾ inch strips. Dip in honey mustard mix. Then roll in crushed corn flakes and put on cookie sheet.

Bake for 10 to 15 minutes or until done.

PER SERVING: 25 CALORIES (KCAL); TRACE TOTAL FAT; (16% CALORIES FROM FAT); 1G PROTEIN; 5G CARBOHYDRATE; 0MG CHOLESTEROL; 175MG SODIUM

"My kids loved these! They said these are better than Kentucky Fried Chicken's and asked if we could have this again next week!" —Lori Sparks

Great Lunch Box Tricks
Some Hip Tips to Help You Pack it Right

Having your child take her own lunch is probably one of the healthiest things a parent can do for their school aged children. Those horrible preservative-packed, lunchlike "meals" that are found in the cheese section of the grocery store, would definitely not qualify as taking a lunch.

Like anything else, lunch is a time to balance out again and it's important that your child has a decent protein/carbo ratio, to get her through the rest of her day. I love the Ultimate Tortilla Roll-Ups (*page 160*) for a lunch box—they're quite easy to make, pack very well and kids love them. There are hundreds of variations on a theme, too. You don't have to just stick with any one recipe—tortillas make great transportation for any filling. Experiment a little bit and try different things.

There are also a few recipes for tasty, packable dips to go with the healthy chips in this cookbook, if having chips in your child's lunch box is a big deal. Just throw a little hummus or something in a Tupperware container and threaten to give your child a ration of only bread and water if they don't bring home the container. A couple of veggies for that already-packed dip isn't hard, either.

I love packing bananas in lunch boxes, although almost any fruit will do. Bananas are easy, convenient, a great source of potassium and come in their own carrying case. Pack it on the very top though, and wrap it a couple of napkins for protection.

This book has a couple of recipes for cookies and recipes for Puffy Grain Bars and Retro Granola bars that also pack well. Toss it in a bag, and you have your own nifty version of those supposed "healthy" nutri-whatever bars. *Cool Fruits* also has great packable lunch box stuff (see resources).

You know how I am about water drinking and I make no exceptions when it comes to packing lunches. I think the smartest move you can make is freezing a water bottle (size will depend on the size of the lunch box) and using that to keep the lunch box cold. By the time lunch rolls around, the water has thawed and it has served two purposes: hydrating your child and keeping his lunch cold, without having to deal with one of those goofy blue ice thingies that leak blue stuff everywhere.

Packing a lunch isn't a big deal and something you can easily train your child to do. Allowing your child free range in a school cafeteria is hazardous to her health, unless they can make good choices. That is, if there even are good choices available.

Emergency Dinner!

Everyone needs a whole repertoire of Emergency Dinners. This one gets two thumbs way up from my kids!

Servings: 3

2 ¼ cups brown rice, use Uncle Ben's Instant variety unless you have some already cooked on hand. IF that is so, this isn't a real emergency, is it?

15 ounces black beans, canned, drained

¼ cup cheddar cheese, low-fat, shredded

Cook rice according to directions. Heat beans.

Dole out three bowls and divvy it all up and serve. Top with cheese, salsa, and low-fat sour cream. If you've got time, warm some tortillas to go with it...talk about living la Vida loca.

PER SERVING: 652 CALORIES (KCAL); 6G TOTAL FAT; (7% CALORIES FROM FAT); 21G PROTEIN; 127G CARBOHYDRATE; 2MG CHOLESTEROL; 499MG SODIUM

Fast and Easy Crazy Y2K Bean Stew

Got a couple of cans of beans in your Y2K stockpile? This will help diminish the ranks some and will take you 15 minutes to make—tops, depending on how fast you are with a can opener.

Serves 6

2 carrots, chopped
1 celery, chopped
1 onion, chopped
4 cans beans, assorted, your choice
4 cans chicken broth
2 cans diced tomatoes
1 teaspoon thyme
1 teaspoon garlic powder

In a large saucepan, sauté onion, carrot and celery in 1 tablespoon of oil till wilted. Add chicken broth.

Add drained beans and canned tomatoes, season and simmer for 10 minutes. Ta Da! There's dinner!

PER SERVING: 518 CALORIES (KCAL); 3G TOTAL FAT; (4% CALORIES FROM FAT); 35G PROTEIN; 91G CARBOHYDRATE; 0MG CHOLESTEROL; 547MG SODIUM

"In words of all the grandchildren DELICIOUSSSSSSSSSSSSSSSSSSSSSSSSS. You called it crazy bean stew, so for the three cans of beans I used pinto, butter beans, and chili beans. It was really good. In my own words, "This is the easiest and most delicious stew I have eaten."
—Sharon Peters

Fast and Furious Chicken and Rice
or Arroz con pollo rapido

Fast and furious recipes like this are lifelines when you have absolutely zero time.

Serves 4

4 boneless, skinless chicken breasts
1 teaspoon garlic powder
1 teaspoon cumin
1 jar salsa
½ can chicken broth
2 cups brown rice, cooked, if you don't have cooked on hand, make instant brown rice.

Preheat oven to 375 degrees.

In a 9 x 13 pan, place frozen chicken breasts and sprinkle with seasonings. Spoon half a jar of salsa on top of the breasts, and pour ½ can chicken broth in the pan. Bake for 20 minutes or until done.

In the meantime, prepare rice according to directions.

When chicken is done, cut horizontally and serve on top of rice with more salsa and low-fat sour cream.

PER SERVING: 415 CALORIES (KCAL); 7G TOTAL FAT; (16% CALORIES FROM FAT); 56G PROTEIN; 28G CARBOHYDRATE; 144MG CHOLESTEROL; 503MG SODIUM

"The Fast and Easy chicken was very good and easy. You'll want to double this recipe. Everyone will want a second helping." —Debbie Martin

Righteous Rice

If there was such a thing as McRice's, you might see a sign proudly displayed saying, "Over 1.5 billion served." The fact is, rice is the staple food for a substantial percentage of people in the world everyday.

Most of us grew up consuming white rice or something along the lines of a "San Francisco treat". The nutritional wonder of brown rice was either unknown or relegated to the weirdo, tie-dyed, hippie crowd. Even the accessibility of good brown rice was somewhat dubious. The grocery stores weren't cooperating and the closest thing to brown rice might be a stale bag stuck on the bottom shelf somewhere.

But no longer. With its wondrous nutritional qualities being touted by nutrition gurus, rice has finally begun to show up, front and center, on the menu. Good quality, nutrient-dense brown rice has finally wrangled an invitation to the party and brought a few friends and relatives, too.

But before you let just the plain wrap, brown rice in, a few of his companions and relatives are also worthy of consideration:

• **Short grain**—this is a sticky-type rice, perfect for the base of a stir fry or anything that you have heaped over the top. It's a little chewy, but easily maneuverable—from fork to mouth—especially for kids.

• **Long grain**—this is a lighter, fluffier rice, with the grains remaining separate when they are cooked. Great for a pilaf or a side dish.

• **Basmati**—much like a long grain rice, it is light and fluffy, but has a distinctive perfume that smells just heavenly when it is cooking. The flavor is wonderful, though not as pronounced as the aroma.

• **Jasmine**—this is another aromatic rice, like basmati, that smells sort of flowery when cooking, but the flavor is more that of regular long grain rice.

• **Sweet brown rice**—this is a short grain rice with a higher starch and sugar content. You could use this product in rice pudding recipes, but it isn't necessary.

• **Wild rice**—as wonderful and flavorful as wild rice is, it isn't a rice at all. It is the seed of an aquatic grass that is related to the rice family.

• **Quinoa**—pronounced, keen-wa, is also not a rice. It is an ancient grain, just rediscovered and enjoying it's place in the limelight. Packed with nutrients, it's used similarly to rice.

While this is by no means an exhaustive list—there are many, many types of brown rice on the market today, it is certainly a good beginning. The only thing essential is that it is brown; that's where the nutrients and the fiber are, the type is up to you and your imagination of what could be done with it.

French Fries

These are just fabulous. Everyone loves these at my house. What's not to like? They're easy, fast and delicious.
Serves 4

4 russet potatoes, scrubbed
1 tablespoon safflower oil
salt, pepper, garlic powder to taste

Preheat oven to 425 degrees.

Slice clean potatoes into steak fries and place in a mixing bowl. Drizzle oil over the top and shake on the seasoning. Toss with clean hands, then place carefully on to a cookie sheet. Make sure the fries aren't laying on top of each other.

Bake for 10 minutes, take out of the oven and turn over. Bake another 10 minutes, then remove to a serving plate.

PER SERVING: 89 CALORIES (KCAL); 3G TOTAL FAT; (34% CALORIES FROM FAT); 2G PROTEIN; 13G CARBOHYDRATE; 0MG CHOLESTEROL; 5MG SODIUM

"We tried this recipe tonight and it got a 10 from everyone!!! They want more tomorrow.
I did have to add a little extra oil. maybe my taters were bigger than yours.
I think this was just as easy as making those frozen ones from the store and much better." —Polly

Hamburger Soup

Mom made, kid approved, easy, easy tasty soup.
Serves 10

1 pound ground beef, extra lean
garlic powder, salt and pepper to taste
1 onion, minced
1 cup diced tomatoes, canned
1 cup frozen peas, I use petite peas, much
**   better than those big tough old things**
5 cups chicken broth
2 cups whole wheat pasta, fuscilli or shells,
**   barely cooked**

Cook beef, seasoning it liberally with garlic, pepper and a little salt. Drain any visible grease. Add minced onion and cook till onion is wilted.

Add the rest of the ingredients and simmer till shells and onion are both done.

Season and serve.

For fun, lose the pasta and serve instead like a stew on garlic mashed potatoes.

PER SERVING: 145 CALORIES (KCAL); 9G TOTAL FAT; (54% CALORIES FROM FAT); 12G PROTEIN; 4G CARBOHYDRATE; 31MG CHOLESTEROL; 430MG SODIUM

"Normally, I don't like leftovers but I loved Hamburger Soup till it was gone.
I want mom to make it again soon." —Ryan McGuinn, age 10

Hash-it-out

Great way to use up healthy leftovers and make a high quality protein meal at the same time.
Serves 4

2 potatoes, baked and chopped
1 onion, chopped
4 egg whites
4 eggs
8 ounces tofu, firm, Process tofu in food
    processor to resemble cottage cheese, or
    use leftover meat, vegetables, whatever
    you have on hand instead of the tofu or
    in addition to the tofu
½ teaspoon thyme
2 tablespoons safflower oil
¼ red bell pepper , chopped (optional)
¼ green bell pepper, chopped (optional)

Heat 1 tablespoon of oil in a large skillet. Add onion and sauté till wilted. Add potato and the rest of the oil. Continue cooking till browned. Add tofu, thyme and salt and pepper to taste.

Add eggs and move the whole mess around like scrambled eggs. Or not. Some like it to set up like an omelet. I don't like it that way.

Serve good and hot. You could top with cheese if you like. Actually, you could do anything you want with this. See what our testers did!

PER SERVING: 247 CALORIES (KCAL); 14G TOTAL FAT; (49% CALORIES FROM FAT); 15G PROTEIN; 16G CARBOHYDRATE; 187MG CHOLESTEROL; 119MG SODIUM

"This was good—I added some red and green bell pepper, I think that gives it some oomph and color."
—Carol Kimbrough

"Excellent! I made it with mushrooms and included the green pepper and red pepper.
The kids loved it topped with a little shredded cheese, Kenny and I loved it with salsa!"
—Nita Crabb

Just Like Mama's Mashed Potatoes

Low in fat, with just a tiny bit of butter on the top. You'll love these!
Serves 4

4 potatoes, peeled and quartered
1 quart water
2 teaspoons garlic powder
salt and pepper
4 ounces low-fat cream cheese
½ cup milk, low-fat

Place the peeled potatoes in a pot and cover with water. Boil till very tender, drain. Add remaining ingredients and take out your aggression on your poor potatoes with a real, old fashioned potato masher. *Don't* use a mixer unless you want glutinous potatoes resembling wallpaper paste. Season to taste. Top with the tiniest amount of butter, just to get the feel of it, without turning it into hip food.

PER SERVING: 179 CALORIES (KCAL); 5G TOTAL FAT; (26% CALORIES FROM FAT); 7G PROTEIN; 26G CARBOHYDRATE; 17MG CHOLESTEROL; 228MG SODIUM

"The potatoes were 'Just like Mama's' indeed.
I'm currently on a diet and with the use of low-fat cream cheese they fit into my eating plan
and made me feel like I was cheating all at once!"—Judy Toney

Leanne's Lazy Lasagna

Making lasagna shouldn't require expert hand/eye coordination just to have a decent meal.
You know what I'm talking about if you have ever put the ricotta on the cooked noodles and tried laying
them straight in the casserole.

Serves 10

16 ounces noodles, your choice, cooked al dente
28 ounces spaghetti sauce, whatever you have on hand
6 ounces cottage cheese, low-fat
½ pound ground beef, extra lean
½ pound mozzarella cheese, part skim milk, shredded
1 tablespoon Paul Prudhomme Pizza and Pasta seasoning
3 teaspoons garlic powder
1 tablespoon basil

Preheat oven to 350 degrees. Drain and cool noodles. Set aside.

Brown ground beef, seasoning with salt and pepper.

Drain off all grease. Blot well with paper towels.

In a mixing bowl, add everything but the mozzarella and mix like mad.

Slosh this mess into your prepared casserole dish and top with the cheese.

Bake about 30 minutes, till nice and warm, but don't brown the cheese.

COOKING NOTES: Feel free to add more cheese...if dairy is an issue, process some tofu in a food processor till it resembles cottage cheese, add a little garlic powder and dried basil—it's wonderful! Heck, you might even want to just use tofu and not tell anyone. It adds a wonderful flavor and texture...and you know me, I'm no tofu fan so I wouldn't steer you wrong!

PER SERVING: 392 CALORIES (KCAL); 14G TOTAL FAT; (31% CALORIES FROM FAT); 21G PROTEIN; 47G CARBOHYDRATE; 72MG CHOLESTEROL; 607MG SODIUM

"Since this recipe has my name in it, I figured I could 'really' be lazy—so I asked my 12-year-old daughter, Rachel, to prepare it. She said it was easy to put together, and the family thinks it's molto bene!" —Lee Ann Roberts

Mashed Potato Soup

Can't get any easier than this! If you have children, saddle them up to the potato peeler and let 'em have at it.

Serves 4

1 great big pot of mashed potatoes (about 4 cups)
2 cups chicken broth
1 cup milk
grated cheddar cheese (low-fat)

Make mashed potatoes. Add chicken broth and milk. Bring to an *almost* boil. (You don't want to see cream soups separate—it'll make you cry, and that'll happen if you boil any milk based soup or sauce.)

Stir it up. Then serve it up. Top with a little cheddar cheese. Or more if you're feeling kinda cheesy.

PER SERVING: 227 CALORIES (KCAL); 11G TOTAL FAT; (44% CALORIES FROM FAT); 18G PROTEIN; 13G CARBOHYDRATE; 33MG CHOLESTEROL; 1646MG SODIUM

"I looked on your web site with your articles and found this great easy recipe for potato soup! That is another one of those recipes I have been looking for, thank you —it was so good!"—Lori Sparks

Not Your Mother's Tuna Casserole

Lynn Nelson of the BusyCooks site (http://busycooks.about.com) had a contest about three years ago called, "Not Your Mother's Tuna Casserole" recipe contest. I was feeling lucky (sheepish, actually) and surprise—I won.

Serves 4

1 box white cheddar macaroni and cheese
½ onion, chopped
1 can albacore tuna, drained
½ tablespoon unsalted butter
1/8 cup unsalted butter
1 cup skim milk
1 cup saltine cracker crumbs
¾ cup cheddar cheese, low-fat, shredded

Boil water to make boxed mac and cheese. Cook pasta and drain.

In the meantime, chop your onion, open and drain your tuna and get ready to launch into tuna casserole land.

In a medium-sized skillet, melt your measly ½ tablespoon of butter. (I'm trying to be good about the butter, but sometimes I slip a little extra in) Sauté your onion and as it turns clear, add the drained tuna. Now add the milk, butter and sauce packet from the box and cook till it thickens. Schlep everything together except the saltines and cheddar and stick it in a greased 2-quart casserole dish. Top with saltines and then cheese. Bake for about 15 minutes, give or take, in a preheated 350 degree oven.

If you are like me, you will be a) blown away that something so easy could taste so good b) make it so often everyone eventually begins to groan c) sneak the leftovers for lunch before the kids find out.

COOKING NOTES: Make *sure* you only use solid white albacore tuna. That cheapie stuff smells like cat food when you open the can. If it smells like cat food...well....

PER SERVING: 216 CALORIES (KCAL); 11G TOTAL FAT; (46% CALORIES FROM FAT); 9G PROTEIN; 19G CARBOHYDRATE; 25MG CHOLESTEROL; 430MG SODIUM

Pizza Muffins

Quick and easy lunch for kids.
Serves 2

2 English muffins, mixed grain, split in half
½ cup spaghetti sauce
½ cup mozzarella cheese, part skim milk, shredded

Preheat oven to 400 degrees. Split muffins and place on cookie sheet in oven for as many minutes as it takes you to grate ½ cup of mozzarella cheese.

Next, top muffin halves with sauce and cheese and bake at 400 degrees for 10 minutes.

You can add just about anything to you want besides the sauce and cheese. Your choice!

PER SERVING: 302 CALORIES (KCAL); 9G TOTAL FAT; (26% CALORIES FROM FAT); 15G PROTEIN; 41G CARBOHYDRATE; 15MG CHOLESTEROL; 732MG SODIUM

Poor Tater Supper

Potatoes baked and stuffed—just that simple.
Serves 4

4 Idaho potatoes, baked
2 cups vegetables, your choice, sautéed or
whatever. Or do what I do and use what-
ever you have on hand and empty out
your Tupperware from the fridge.
8 ounces cottage cheese, low-fat
¼ cup chicken broth
½ cup cheddar cheese, low-fat, shredded

Preheat oven to 400 degrees. Wash, pierce and bake potatoes for an hour. You should use good-sized potatoes. Remember, this is dinner.

Split potatoes lengthwise and place innards into a large bowl. Mix well with veggies, cottage cheese and chicken broth, season liberally with salt and pepper. Stuff potato back in the skin and top with cheddar.

Bake till bubbly, about 15 minutes.

PER SERVING: 164 CALORIES (KCAL); 2G TOTAL FAT; (9% CALORIES FROM FAT); 13G PROTEIN; 24G CARBOHYDRATE; 5MG CHOLESTEROL; 372MG SODIUM

"A lovely change of pace for baked potatoes, and so pretty, too"—Christina Fredricks

Quick Quinoa Lasagna

Vickilynn strikes again! This time, with a delicious lasagna recipe.
Serves 12

1-15oz. can tomatoes
2-8oz. cans tomato sauce
1 teaspoon sea salt
2 teaspoons oregano
1 cup onion, minced
3 cloves garlic, crushed
¼ cup olive oil
1 pound ground beef, extra lean
3 cups quinoa, cooked, see cooking notes on quinoa pilaf for important notes on preparation.
½ pound ricotta cheese, part skim milk
¼ pound mozzarella cheese, part skim milk
¼ pound parmesan cheese or use Romano cheese

In a large pan, light sauté onion and garlic in olive oil until soft, but do not brown. In another pan, brown ground meat and drain fat. Add cooked meat to the onion and garlic mixture and heat briefly. Add tomato sauce, tomatoes, salt and oregano. Reduce heat and gently simmer.

Preheat oven to 350 degrees.

In a 9 x 13 pan, place a thin layer of the sauce, following with a layer of quinoa and a layer of cheeses. Repeat this pattern ending with sauce and extra parmesan cheese on top. Bake uncovered for about 35 minutes. Remove from the oven and let stand 5-10 minutes before cutting.

COOKING NOTES: Quinoa must be thoroughly rinsed to remove the outside bitter coating. See complete directions on Quinoa Pilaf recipe on *page 117*.

PER SERVING: 325 CALORIES (KCAL); 14G TOTAL FAT; (22% CALORIES FROM FAT); 16G PROTEIN; 35G CARBOHYDRATE; 25MG CHOLESTEROL; 589MG SODIUM

"I'm a homemaker and mother of six. I try to feed my children the healthiest meals I can. However, I would not have tried a recipe like the Quick Quinoa Lasagna on my own. It really was delicious! We enjoyed it and I plan to make it again!" —Kimberly Halbert

Quinoa Pilaf

Popular guest columnist, Vickilynn Haycraft often introduces new whole foods on my ezine "Healthy-Foods".
Here's her recipe for Quinoa Pilaf from her column, "What's THAT?" from the Healthy-Foods newsletter.
Serves 12

½ **cup carrot, diced**
½ **cup onion, diced**
½ **cup celery, diced**
½ **cup sweet red pepper, diced**
6 **cups quinoa, cooked**
1 **teaspoon unsalted butter**
2 **cloves garlic, crushed**
¼ **cup almonds, sliced**
¼ **teaspoon oregano**

Sauté chopped veggies in butter until crisp-tender. Add oregano. Add sautéed veggies to cooked hot quinoa, mixing well. Add salt to taste. Dry roast almonds in a heavy skillet until lightly golden. Add almonds and mix.

Serving Ideas : Just in case you didn't think about it, you *could* easily substitute brown rice. Long grained brown rice works best.

COOKING NOTES: Quinoa (keen-wa) is an ancient grain that can be easily used in recipes calling for rice or other grains. To make, soak and wash the quinoa to remove the outer coating of the grain. This is an important step——otherwise anything you make with the quinoa will be bitter. To cook, bring 2 cups of water to a boil and add 1 cup rinsed quinoa and bring to a boil again. Cover and reduce heat and cook until grains are translucent and fluffy, about 15 minutes.

PER SERVING: 346 CALORIES (KCAL); 7G TOTAL FAT; (17% CALORIES FROM FAT); 12G PROTEIN; 61G CARBOHYDRATE; 1MG CHOLESTEROL; 25MG SODIUM

"This was a very satisfying dish to make...it turned out so pretty!! —Tracey Kirch

Tunisian Cous Cous

*Chef Henri taught me how to make this years ago. I have since revamped it somewhat,
but it's a huge favorite around here. 4 Servings*

**1 ½ cups couscous, use whole wheat
couscous from the health food store**
2 cups chicken broth
1 teaspoon cumin
1 teaspoon garlic

In a pot, bring chicken broth to a boil. Add couscous, spices and stir. Feel free to rev up the spices if you like—I certainly don't add such minuscule amounts. I'm just trying to be conservative here for the sake of uninitiated taste buds. Remove from heat and let sit for about 10-15 minutes. Fluff with a fork and serve.

PER SERVING: 266 CALORIES (KCAL); 1G TOTAL FAT; (4% CALORIES FROM FAT); 11G PROTEIN; 51G CARBOHYDRATE; 0MG CHOLESTEROL; 389MG SODIUM

White Chili

This was big in the 80's——I think mainly because it was sort of a dished-up version of Nouvelle Cuisine. Remember that? Big plate, tiny drop of food artfully displayed? Well, this recipe stands the test of time.

Serves 8

2 pounds boneless, skinless chicken breasts

2 onions, chopped

2 ½ cups chicken broth, canned or home-made

1 can green chilies, chopped

1 can tomatillos

2 teaspoons each: cumin and garlic powder

1 teaspoon oregano

3 cups white beans, cooked, canned or make yourself

½ bunch cilantro, chopped—optional

1 pound low-fat jack cheese, grated

In a large saucepan, heat a small amount of oil and sauté the onion. When the onion is translucent, add chicken. Cook for a couple of minutes, max. Don't let it stick and don't add a ton of oil to keep it cooking either.

Add everything else, except the cilantro and cheese. If you want, after sautéing the chicken and onion together, you could finish the recipe in a crock pot. If you do, cook on high for about 3 hours or so. If you want it to cook all day, put it on low. You just need to get it nice and hot. If you are doing this on the stove top, simmer for about 20 minutes.

Serve in nice big bowls, sprinkle with cilantro if you like, and some grated cheese. Served with buttermilk cornbread and a big salad, this is a wonderful, yummy meal.

PER SERVING: 254 CALORIES (KCAL); 4G TOTAL FAT; (13% CALORIES FROM FAT); 34G PROTEIN; 20G CARBOHYDRATE; 69MG CHOLESTEROL; 304MG SODIUM

"White Chili—warming, filling and just the right spice; it smells sooo good while it simmers in the crockpot."—Sue LeMay

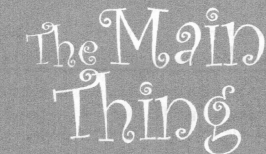

The Main Thing

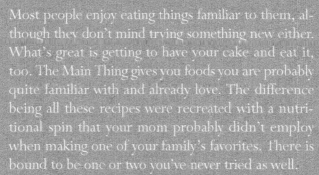

Most people enjoy eating things familiar to them, although they don't mind trying something new either. What's great is getting to have your cake and eat it, too. The Main Thing gives you foods you are probably quite familiar with and already love. The difference being all these recipes were recreated with a nutritional spin that your mom probably didn't employ when making one of your family's favorites. There is bound to be one or two you've never tried as well.

   Have fun and keep cooking—I bet you a nickel one or two of these recipes gets jotted down on a 3x5 and passed on to your sister-in-law.

Chicken Pot Pie

This is the Mother of all mama foods—comfort food that totally hits the spot, especially on a cold, winter night. The flavor is greatly improved by baking the chicken and deglazing the pan, but any cooked chicken will work.

Serves 10

5 cups chicken, cooked and chopped
1 onion, medium sized, chopped
3 carrots, chopped
½ celery stalk, minced
¾ cup frozen peas, use petite peas, big diff.
2 cups chicken broth, homemade or
   canned
2 tablespoons whole wheat pastry flour
2 tablespoons unsalted butter
1 teaspoon garlic powder
2 teaspoons thyme
salt and pepper, to taste
½ recipe of whole wheat pastry crust *(page 186)*

In a large skillet, melt 1 tablespoon of the butter (or more if you need it) and sauté onion, carrot and celery all together for about 5 minutes, till they are wilted.

Salt and pepper to taste.

Add chicken to the mixture and toss well. Season with garlic and thyme. Pour into a bowl and set aside. In the same skillet melt the remaining butter, add flour and whisk over medium heat for about 3 minutes. Add chicken stock and cook, constantly whisking it in the pan until thickened.

Pour gravy over the top of chicken mixture and mix well. Add frozen peas and mix again.

In a 9 x13 pan, pour chicken mixture and top with crust. Make some slits for steam to escape.

Bake for 20 to 30 minutes in preheated 375 degree oven. Watch your crust—when it's browned nicely (not too brown—it will continue to cook a minute or two once it comes out of the oven) pull it out.

PER SERVING: 236 CALORIES (KCAL); 16G TOTAL FAT; (62% CALORIES FROM FAT); 17G PROTEIN; 5G CARBOHYDRATE; 84MG CHOLESTEROL; 234MG SODIUM

"Your instructions on the chicken pot pie made it very easy, sometimes cookbooks make it sound to hard so you don't even want to try. It is refreshing to see easy instructions with basic ingredients. The smell of this cooking is absolutely heavenly. It takes a while to make, but it is worth every second of it!! Your family will love you for this one, mine sure did!" —Lori Sparks

COOKING NOTES: Make sure you mince the celery. People get hostile when they get gargantuan hunks of celery in their pot pies. Celery chunks remind me of the days when my mom would open up a can of chop suey when she and my dad would go out. There were four huge hunks of celery, some frightening looking bean sprouts and the rest of it was water chestnuts. I am lucky I lived to tell about it.

Deglazing a pan involves adding water to a pan that has cooked chicken and there is drippings and stuck stuff on the bottom of it. That stuff is cooking gold and adds unbelievable flavor to whatever you are cooking. You should get into a habit of always deglazing your pan and adding that to your chicken broth. For example, in this recipe, if you had about a cup of deglazed liquid, you could add reduce the amount of chicken broth by half and use half chicken broth and half deglazed liquid. *(for more on deglazing, see Cooking Basics)*

Crock Roast

Pot roast is pot roast until you've had Crock Roast. Bet your mom's never tasted this good.

Serves 10

3 pounds rump roast, trimmed
3 cloves garlic
1 teaspoon sea salt
2 teaspoons thyme
1 onion, quartered
4 carrot, sliced 1" thick
1 cup red wine
½ cup beef broth

In a large skillet, brown the beef on high on all sides. Salt and pepper to taste.

Place beef in the crockpot and top with the thyme, and onion. Put carrots around the side.

In the skillet that browned the beef, add broth and red wine and cook till boiling, deglazing the pan as you go. Pour this on top of the beef.

Place lid on the crockpot and cook on high for about 4 - 5 hours.

PER SERVING: 227 CALORIES (KCAL); 7G TOTAL FAT; (29% CALORIES FROM FAT); 31G PROTEIN; 5G CARBOHYDRATE; 79MG CHOLESTEROL; 356MG SODIUM

"Oooh la la! One bite of this tender, juicy roast and I felt as if I had been transported to a little cafe somewhere in the south of France. Now, if only I knew how to say "Excellent!" or something of that sort in French, I would end my quote with it!" —Lee Ann Roberts

Crockpot Taco Meat

This is definitely something you want to come home to after a long day away from home.
Serves 10 or more

3 pounds beef bottom round
1 tablespoon cumin
1 tablespoon garlic powder
2 teaspoons oregano
1 teaspoon sea salt

Brown the beef in a big skillet with a little bit of oil, cook it on a medium high heat with a little salt and pepper, just to get it browned nicely. Transfer it to your crockpot.

Toss together spices in a small bowl and set aside.

Deglaze the skillet with 1 cup of water, vigorously attacking the pot with your wire whisk. When the water boils and reduces by half, pour over the top of the roast.

Sprinkle half your seasoning on the top of your roast. Put the lid on and turn on low and cook for 8 hours. Meat should be shredding nicely when it's done.

Let cool and shred meat with a fork. Place in a bowl, sprinkle remaining seasoning and cover and let sit to allow flavors to meld. Prepare the rest of your meal.

COOKING NOTES: Serve with warmed tortillas, cheese, rice, beans, shredded lettuce, cilantro, chopped tomatoes, onions...whatever your little heart desires! This is a good basic for whatever Mexican dish you like—easy or more involved. It's your choice!

I make black beans and serve with this. Having beans will help cut back on copious amounts of meat consumption. Make a pot of brown rice, too and serve with warmed tortillas, shredded, low-fat cheese, no fat sour cream, salsa, cilantro—whatever turns your key. This is an easy-to-make dinner that could easily become another night of dinner if you prepare the beans and rice to go with it.

PER SERVING: 269 CALORIES (KCAL); 15G TOTAL FAT; (52% CALORIES FROM FAT); 30G PROTEIN; 1G CARBOHYDRATE; 95MG CHOLESTEROL; 240MG SODIUM

"The Crockpot Taco Meat mix was a big hit here. The meat was moist and tender and very easy to prepare. The flavor was a nice change from the 'brown ground beef and dump on a packet of store bought mix' taco filling that tends to be all too common here. The quantity of meat the recipe prepared is sufficient for us to have two more taco meals. This one is a keeper at this household. It was easy to prepare and very tasty. The only hard part was keeping the kids out of the crockpot to see what smelled so good!"
—Tammi Klusewitz

Mexican Seasoning

Those envelopes of taco seasoning are expensive and have stuff you don't want, like MSG (sometimes called "natural flavoring"). Here's an inexpensive alternative and much healthier, too.
Servings: 1 batch.

1/3 cup chili powder
¼ cup cumin
4 teaspoons crushed red pepper, (totally optional, depends on your family's heat tolerance)
1 tablespoon oregano
1/8 cup garlic powder
1 tablespoon onion powder

Mix all together and store in a sealed container or ziptop bag.

Double Duty Chicken

This is the crockpot way to delectable chicken for any recipe and a killer chicken stock for any soup. It takes almost no effort to cook this up and it's a great thing to stock your freezer with.

Serves 12

1 roasting chicken
1 onion
1 carrot
1 celery rib
4 cloves garlic
1 teaspoon thyme
salt and pepper, to taste

Wash and dry chicken and place in crockpot. Break whole carrot and celery in half and place in the cavity of the chicken. Cut the onion in half and stuff into the cavity along with the garlic. It's time to party in the chicken. Don't add any water. Turn on high and cook for about 4 hours. You should have a heavenly smell coming from your kitchen, tender chicken and double rich chicken broth.

When the chicken has cooled, debone, degrease and skin it and chop. Use for a recipe or put it in a bag and freeze.

Strain chicken broth and place in a pot and refrigerate for a few hours. Take the congealed fat off the top and discard. Use broth for a recipe or freeze for future use.

COOKING NOTES: Use this recipe as a starting place to make Shepherd's Pie #1, Chicken Pot Pie or a chicken version of Enchilasgna. The wonderful stock this makes could be easily frozen for use in one of the many soup recipes in this book. Also, there is less fat in this than the recipe says because you have taken all the fat off the top when preparing.

PER SERVING: 249 CALORIES (KCAL); 18G TOTAL FAT; (27% CALORIES FROM FAT); 19G PROTEIN; 2G CARBOHYDRATE; 81MG CHOLESTEROL; 81MG SODIUM

"I cooked this yesterday and today we had it for supper. It was very yummy. What I did was to make a gravy/white sauce from the drippings like you use for chicken and biscuits. Then we heated up the chicken in the microwave. We served the chicken with the French fries and the creamy gravy. Everyone gave it a 10 too!!! That's not an easy task with this family."—Polly

Spice Primer

- ANISE—I never use this, but if you insist on having spices in alphabetical order, you need to start somewhere. Use it in stews, cakes, fish...the list is endless. Whatever turns your key.

- BAY LEAF—Used in stews, soup and great with pot roast. Go easy. Bay leaves are strong. I only use ½ a leaf in my stews.

- BASIL—Ah, the taste of summer. Who can resist fresh basil and tomatoes from the garden tossed with olive oil and garlic on a plate full of pasta? Dried, it is wonderful in soups, pasta dishes and chicken.

- CAYENNE—hot, hot, hot...but good for what ails you, too. Capsicum, the plant it comes from, is used by herbalists for a whole host of maladies.

- CHERVIL—Rhymes with gerbil. Sort of licorice-y tasting with parsley overtones. Why not just use anise and parsley and keep your lazy susan cleared of stuff you'll never use.

- DILL—It's not just for pickles. Try some dill sprinkled on fish, chicken or even in a light cream soup.

- GARLIC—nectar of the gods, well, bulb of the gods anyway. Garlic has a way of making the most ordinary food gourmet. Try sprinkling garlic powder (not garlic salt) into a prepared box of white cheddar macaroni and cheese. Surprise! It's pretty good. Fresh, though, is best. Squeeze it from a press into almost anything.

- GINGER—this is my current flavor of the month. Sprinkle it in your stir-fry, try it on some baked chicken breasts with a little soy sauce and garlic. See the Glossary for more info on working with fresh ginger.

- NUTMEG—I love nutmeg. If you can find nutmeg nuts and the grater that comes with it, buy it. Once you've had freshly grated nutmeg, the powdered stuff in the jar is beneath you. Obviously an ingredient in baking, it's also good grated on sautéed squash, green beans, and carrots.

- OREGANO—A staple in Italian cooking, it's also good in stews and salad dressings.

- PARSLEY—every coffee shop in America uses parsley as a garnish. It's also good for indigestion and bad breath.

- SAGE—think Thanksgiving. Turkey wouldn't be the same without a liberal sprinkling of sage in the stuffing.

- ROSEMARY—spike a roast with garlic and fresh rosemary, and you'll never be the same. Aromatic and wonderful.

- THYME—I use this a lot in recipes. It's strong and adds a hint of character to an otherwise pretty standard dish. Use it with chicken, soups and beef.

- VANILLA—make sure you get pure vanilla extract, and not vanillin which is fake-o and gross. Pure vanilla adds a whole dimension to just about anything.

This is quite an abbreviated list of spices, but it's a good start. I've skipped a lot of them because they are used so infrequently and just take up room on the lazy susan. Besides, who cares what turmeric is used for anyway? I can't even pronounce it.

Enchilasagna

What do you get when you cross a lasagna with an enchilada? Give up? Follow this recipe and you'll find out!
Serves 12

2 10-ounce cans enchilada sauce
1 12-15-ounce can tomato sauce
1 pound ground beef, extra lean, cooked and drained (for fun, use 4 cups cooked and chopped chicken for a different flavor!)
1 tablespoon cumin
1 tablespoon garlic powder
12 corn tortillas, chopped
12 ounces black beans, canned, drained
1 pound low-fat cheddar cheese, or use jack cheese

Preheat oven to 350 degrees and grease a 13x9 pan.

In a saucepan, combine enchilada sauce and tomato sauce. Let simmer.

Brown beef, drain and add seasonings and salt and pepper to taste.

Add about ½ of the sauce to browned beef and set aside.

On the bottom of the pan, pour ¾ cup of sauce and add about 1/3 of the beef mixture and then beans.

Next, make a layer of corn tortillas, using 1/3 of what you have.

Add more beef, 1/3 of the beans, ¼ of the cheese

Repeat these layers: corn tortillas, beef, bean and cheese, till everything is gone. Top with remaining sauce and remaining cheese.

Bake uncovered for 30 to 40 minutes. Wait 10 minutes before digging in!

PER SERVING: 290 CALORIES (KCAL); 14G TOTAL FAT; (22% CALORIES FROM FAT); 20G PROTEIN; 20G CARBOHYDRATE; 46MG CHOLESTEROL; 552MG SODIUM

"This recipe has great flavor! Everyone enjoyed eating it, and I was happy at how easy it was to prepare. I could do parts of the preparation in advance, then assemble the casserole and bake it. This will be a part of our regular rotation from now on."
—Jen Pitoniak

Fajitas Pollo Loca

Seriously good stuff—not a recipe to miss out on. Fire up the barby for extra flavor.

Serves 8

¼ **cup lime juice**
¼ **cup rice wine vinegar**
5 **cloves garlic, pressed**
5 **teaspoons cumin**
2 **tablespoons olive oil**
2 **pounds boneless, skinless chicken breasts**
2 **cups pico de gallo (page 135)**
8 **corn tortillas**
1 **cup onion, sliced**
1 **cup red bell pepper, sliced**
½ **cup green bell pepper**
1 **tablespoon olive oil**

Light the barbeque.

Prepare marinade: mix lime juice, rice wine vinegar, garlic, cumin and olive oil well. Place chicken breasts in marinade for about 10 minutes.

Grill on the barbeque or broil in your oven.

Remove chicken when it's done. In the meantime, heat remaining olive oil in a skillet or flat-bottomed wok and sauté bell peppers and onion till wilted and cooked, but not mush. You don't want smushy vegetables. Diagonally slice chicken and toss in the skillet with peppers and onions. Mix it up and heat through.

Warm tortillas in a dry skillet, quickly moving them over the heat. Place in a basket to be served at the table.

Serve with pico de gallo, sour cream and chopped fresh cilantro.

PER SERVING: 290 CALORIES (KCAL); 12G TOTAL FAT; (38% CALORIES FROM FAT); 28G PROTEIN; 17G CARBOHYDRATE, 69MG CHOLESTEROL; 104MG SODIUM

"I've tried a number of fajitas recipes over the years and this one tasted the closest to what you get in a restaurant. In addition to taste, I like it because I generally have all the ingredients on hand, and if I didn't, substitutions are easy. That makes it nice for a last minute dinner that my husband doesn't realize is last minute. As I was writing that, he called from the kitchen that dinner was sure delicious. This is a great recipe that will undoubtedly become a regular item for us."—Georgia

Manic Meatloaf

Lovely, wonderful, happy little meatloaf. Something you just have to have with mashed potatoes, at least every so often. This meatloaf is so good, all others will taste like airline food from now on. If you're smart, you'll double or even triple this recipe, cook off a few and freeze them. Makes an amazing sandwich for breakfast the next morning.

Serves 12

1 onion, chopped
1 carrot, chopped
½ red bell pepper, chopped
2 cloves garlic, pressed
2 teaspoons cumin
1 teaspoon nutmeg
½ teaspoon white pepper
½ cup ketchup
2 egg whites
½ cup buttermilk
1 cup oatmeal
2 pounds ground beef, extra lean
1 cup bread crumbs, seasoned

Preheat oven to 375 degrees. In a skillet with a little bit of oil, sauté onion, carrot, bell pepper and garlic till translucent. Set aside.

In a large mixing bowl, combine the remaining ingredients. Salt and pepper liberally.

Add sautéed veggies and mix again well. Shape a loaf to look like a model of the Goodyear blimp and bake for about 45 minutes. But check it—your loaf might be thicker or thinner than mine.

Let rest for about 10 minutes or so (while you finish up the mashed potatoes) and remove from pan and place on a plate with paper towels to remove excess grease.

If you're short on time, grease the daylights out of your muffin tin and make mini-meatloaves. This is one time you'll want to skip the cupcake liners, though.

PER SERVING: 268 CALORIES (KCAL); 14G TOTAL FAT; (47% CALORIES FROM FAT); 18G PROTEIN; 17G CARBOHYDRATE; 53MG CHOLESTEROL; 457MG SODIUM

"What's a real comfort food for me? Meatloaf, mashed potatoes and fixin's. MMMMM! Manic Meatloaf!! I am always looking for a good-tasting meatloaf recipe and this one was a Keeper. It had a smooth and slightly sweet flavor that the children (and mom and dad) really enjoyed. We have been eating up the leftovers for sandwiches today and next time I will make a few of these and freeze the extras! Delicious."—Vickilynn Haycraft

Cooking Basics *or* How to Drive without a Map

There are essentials in cooking like any other skill. Getting a good understanding of what constitutes essential know-how will empower the way you cook from here out, not just with these recipes. Here is a quick list of things to know:

- SALT AND PEPPER—if you'll notice, in my recipes I always write "salt and pepper to taste." (Unless of course, the recipe happens to be a dessert of some kind.) Salt brings out the best of whatever it is you're cooking and pepper gives it a little extra "edge". I mentioned before I use sea salt and I'll mention it again—it's a much better alternative than commercial salts, not nearly as harsh, and in my opinion, I think the taste is nicer. Just go easy—a little goes a long way. Pepper should be fresh ground. The stuff in the can doesn't even warrant comment. Get yourself a peppermill and grind it yourself. I never ask you to measure pepper in a recipe—I think that's just plain nuts. Grind it to taste—you're the best judge of what you like best.

- MIRE POIX—this is a French culinary term (pronounced-meer pwah) that refers to a vegetable mixture of carrot, onion and celery. These three vegetables balance out the flavoring of a stock, soup or whatever else it is you are making. The carrot adds the sweet, the onion the tart and the celery the salt. I call them the culinary trilogy—easier than trying to fake a French accent. Keep these three little ingredients in mind when cooking—they really will make a difference in almost anything you make. I keep the ratio 2:1. Twice the amount of carrot and onion, to celery.

- STOCK—I have given you two great recipes for rich stock, the Double Duty Chicken recipe will reap a most delightful chicken stock thanks to your indentured servant, the crockpot, and the Roast Vegetable stock is also quite good and does the trick in a vegetarian sort of way. Obviously, use these stocks in soups and sauces, but take it a step further and rev up your rice pilaf by cooking the rice in stock or extending a sauce. It's really not too tough to stock a freezer with stock (pardon the obvious pun) and is pretty helpful to have on hand.

- DEGLAZE—this is a term bandied about when talking about making a sauce or gravy. All it means is, add water and scrape all those browned bits of stuff up off the pan bottom and let it boil. This is what adds the rich flavor and depth. It's not hard to do and will make a huge difference flavor-wise. I go positively berserk when I see someone throw a roasting pan into the sink without the benefit of a good scraping up. All that flavor, down the drain.

Persnickety Picadillo

I have made this for years before discovering that it actually had a name.
Everyone loves this, don't worry about the name...your kids will love both the name and the dish!
Serves 6

3 cups brown rice, cooked, set aside
1 pound ground beef, extra lean
2 onions, chopped
1 red bell pepper, chopped
2 cloves garlic, pressed
1 shot ketchup
2 summer squash, diced (in the winter, substitute sweet potato and sneak a little nutmeg in there, too. It's good!)
2 teaspoons cumin
2 teaspoons oregano
1 can beef broth, low sodium, no msg
salt and pepper to taste

In a large skillet, sauté one of the onions and garlic till translucent. Add ground beef, season with half the spices and salt and pepper. Drain well and set aside.

In a smaller skillet, sauté the remaining onion and bell pepper together for a couple of minutes. Add summer squash, season with salt and pepper and cook till squash is almost done. Dump those veggies into the meat mixture.

In that same skillet, mix together the beef broth and ketchup and bring to a boil. Allow to reduce a bit, about 10 minutes. Add the rest of the seasoning, whisking well to blend and cook another minute.

Put the sauce over the top of your meat mixture and mix well. Heat briefly, just to heat through and serve ladled on top of rice in bowls. If you want to get authentic with Picadillo, add green olives and raisins. The very idea of these garnishes (garni?) is completely nauseating to certain members of this household, but if you want to do Picadillo the way it's done, that's the way they do it, whoever "they" are.

PER SERVING: 329 CALORIES (KCAL); 14G TOTAL FAT; (38% CALORIES FROM FAT); 18G PROTEIN; 33G CARBOHYDRATE; 52MG CHOLESTEROL; 114MG SODIUM

"The picadillo is fabulous!" —Dinah Luevano

Pico de Gallo

Pico de Gallo, means Rooster Beak in Spanish. Now that you have had your Spanish lesson, go make this fabulous salsa!

Serves 8

8 tomatoes, chopped
½ bunch cilantro, washed and dried
1 onion, chopped
1 jalapeno, seeded and diced

Mix all chopped ingredients together, season with sea salt. Cover and let sit an hour or so (don't refrigerate) to allow flavors to meld. Serve with anything, except dessert.

PER SERVING: 43 CALORIES (KCAL); 1G TOTAL FAT; (10% CALORIES FROM FAT); 2G PROTEIN; 9G CARBOHYDRATE; 0MG CHOLESTEROL; 16MG SODIUM

Cooking Note: Warning: Handle jalapeno with extreme care. You may even want to use gloves when handling this pepper. Make sure you wash your hands after making this salsa.

Reyna's Enchilada Verde Casserole

This casserole could bring a grown man to his knees begging for more. You don't have let things get so awkward though. I've made this recipe a lot easier by turning it into a casserole. Same effect, just as delicious.

Serve 8

**6 chicken breasts, boneless and skinless,
    cooked and chopped**
2 onions, chopped
2 cloves garlic, pressed
2 teaspoons cumin
12 corn tortillas
2 cans tomatillos
12 ounces low-fat jack cheese, grated

In a skillet, sauté ½ the onion in about a tablespoon of oil. Cook for 2 minutes and add garlic. Cook another 2 minutes and add chicken and cumin. Mix well, set aside.

In a blender, add the rest of the onion and the two cans of tomatillos, juice and all. Blend like mad.

Preheat your oven to 375 degrees and get out a 9 x 13 casserole dish. Pour about a ½ cup of sauce on the bottom of the pan and begin building your casserole.

Start with a sauce (already said that) tortillas, chicken mixture, little cheese and repeat this pattern till finished. Pour the rest of the sauce evenly over the top and sprinkle remaining cheese over that and bake for approximately 20 minutes or until done. Don't over bake, though. You want it hot and melty, not hard and browned.

COOKING NOTES: Reyna made these delicious enchiladas by frying the tortilla in oil. I have tried doing it without the frying in oil part and they fell apart. Then I tried spraying them with cooking spray, still not a good option. So I decided it would be just as good and a whole lot faster just to chop up the tortillas and skip the enchilada making all together and turn this into another version of enchilasagna. But Reyna gets the credit, this recipe is hers and it's the best!

PER SERVING: 308 CALORIES (KCAL); 6G TOTAL FAT; (17% CALORIES FROM FAT); 42G PROTEIN; 21G CARBOHYDRATE; 108MG CHOLESTEROL; 156MG SODIUM

"We all enjoyed this dish. Yummy and filling! It was very easy to put together." —Tracey Kirch

Rubber Chicken

A great inexpensive, easy to make a basic. You'll love stretching this rubber chicken!
Serves 12

1 roasting chicken, washed and patted dry
(about 3 pounds)
½ celery rib, cut in pieces
1 onion, quartered
1 carrot, cut in 2" pieces
salt, pepper, garlic powder to taste

Day One: Make a roasted chicken. If you don't know how, don't fret, I'll help you. Preheat your oven to 375 degrees and place your clean chicken in a roasting pan, breast side up, with all the veggies placed in the cavity. Season liberally and cook. Baste it if you like. Depending on the size, it will take an hour or so to roast. While the chicken is cooking, use the same veggies and throw the neck in some water to make additional stock for the gravy. Cook it on low. When the chicken is done, the leg should move easily in the socket. Before you make gravy, pour all the cooking juice out from the roaster into a bowl to cool. Put it in the fridge or freezer to encourage the fat to glob up on to the top. Then you can skim off that nasty fat and throw it away. Return the juice without the fat, to the same pan and deglaze your pan (see Cooking Basics). In a small mixing bowl, take a tablespoon of whole wheat pastry flour, about ¾ cup of cool water and make a smooth paste. Heat the cooking juice, add the neck broth and then add your paste. Using your wire whisk, whisk like a crazy lady over fairly high heat till your gravy starts to look like gravy. Remove from heat and serve with Just Like Mama's Mashed Potatoes and lots of vegetables. Remember you want leftovers.

Day Two: On the menu tonight is——Chicken and Bean Burritos! To make, pick all the chicken off the bones and toss it together in a pan with a can of black beans. Add about 1 teaspoon each of garlic powder and cumin (more if you're manic!) and warm it up. In the meantime, get out your fixin's: shredded cheese, salsa, chopped cilantro, sour cream——whatever you like. Warm your tortillas and serve.

Day Three: Take the skeletal remains, and throw it in a pot with a stick of celery, a carrot or two and a big onion. Throw a quart of cold water over the top and bring it to a boil. Let it simmer for an hour or so——till the veggies are mushy. Strain the whole thing (now you can throw out that chicken with a good conscience!) and make whatever soup your little heart desires. There is a whole bunch of them in here to get you going!

PER CHICKEN: 274 CALORIES (KCAL); 19G TOTAL FAT; (30% CALORIES FROM FAT); 22G PROTEIN; TRACE CARBOHYDRATE; 113MG CHOLESTEROL; 91MG SODIUM

"We all enjoyed Day 1. But Day 2 everyone LOVED!!! My family is not a big black bean eater. But they gave me the go ahead to make this scrumptious dinner often!! Yummy!!!" —Tracey Kirch

Shepherd's Pie #1

This is a clever leftover, pretending to be a new dinner! One rule at our house: don't ask, don't tell.

Serve 8

3 cups chicken, cooked and shredded
1 onion, chopped
2 carrots, chopped
1 teaspoon thyme
1 ½ cups gravy, degreased, leftover, add a
    little water if it's not quite enough
3 cups mashed potatoes

Take all the meat off the chicken and chop. Hopefully, you have about 3 cups. This is assuming, of course, that you made Rubber Chicken (see *page 137*) the first night. If you didn't make Rubber Chicken the first night, never mind.

Sauté onion and carrot together in a little bit of oil, when onion is translucent, add chopped chicken and seasonings. Pour leftover gravy over the top and heat and mix. If you don't have any gravy leftover, take one can of broth and bring to a boil in a separate skillet. Take 1 heaping tablespoon of flour and mix with cold water in a separate container till smooth and add to boiling broth. Mix vigorously with a wire whisk trying to avoid lumps. (if you get lumps, try and smoosh them out or strain it) Pour into a 9" pie pan.

Warm mashed potatoes. Add a little bit of milk if too stiff.

Pile potatoes on top on chicken mixture, like you're frosting a cake.

Bake in a preheated oven (375 degrees) for 30 minutes.

COOKING NOTES: If you have enough leftover chicken and mashed potatoes for Day 1 of the Rubber Chicken Adventure, this would be a terrific Day 2 option instead of doing the chicken bean burrito thing.

PER SERVING: 214 CALORIES (KCAL); 12G TOTAL FAT; (50% CALORIES FROM FAT); 13G PROTEIN; 13G CARBOHYDRATE; 60MG CHOLESTEROL; 236MG SODIUM

"Another great recipe! Everyone agreed that it was a nice change and a great way to use leftovers. Even AnnaClaire, the 2 year old who isn't into casseroles and first said, 'I don't like it' before the first bite, finished an entire serving. Now, that's saying something!" —Tammi Klusewitz

Shepherd's Pie #2

Everyone likes this. Easy to make, easy to serve and easy to eat.

Serves 8

1 pound ground beef, extra lean
1 onion, chopped
1 carrot, chopped
½ teaspoon rosemary, crushed
salt and pepper, garlic powder to taste
3 cups mashed potatoes

In a large skillet, add a little oil and sauté vegetables till wilted. Pull from the skillet and set aside. In the meantime, put your potatoes on to boil to make mashed potatoes, unless you have some left over.

Using the same skillet you used for the veggies, crumble beef up into the skillet and sprinkle with garlic powder, rosemary and salt and pepper to taste. Drain fat well. Either make gravy (see directions on Shepherd's Pie #1 and substitute beef broth for chicken broth) or use leftover gravy and pour over ground beef.

Mix ground beef with vegetables and pour into a 9" pie tin. Make mashed potatoes, or warm leftovers and spread over the top of the meat mixture.

Bake in a preheated 375 degree oven for 35 minutes or till nice and hot.

PER SERVING: 204 CALORIES (KCAL); 11G TOTAL FAT; (50% CALORIES FROM FAT); 12G PROTEIN; 12G CARBOHYDRATE; 41MG CHOLESTEROL; 225MG SODIUM

"Another quick and easy success. Leftover mashed potatoes now have a new life in our house. Lacking rosemary, I substituted thyme and enjoyed the results. This will definitely show back up on our table."
—Mary O'Neil

A Tidbit on Tofu

You never heard it from me that tofu is a flavorful, delectable treat. Nope, not even close to it, as a matter of fact. Tofu represents everything bland and banal in this life. However, that doesn't mean it isn't good for you. On the contrary, tofu is amazing stuff, able to leap tall nutritional buildings in a single bound. The thing to know about tofu is how to use it. I use it in things where it is the mere nutritional underpinnings to a dish or drink. A good example of this is smoothies. I use silkened tofu in smoothies all the time—and you would never know it was there were it not for the empty container in the trash. Or whip it up a bit with some parsley and garlic in the food processor to stand in for ricotta in your lasagna. I have even heard tell of tofu cheesecakes being half-decent.

Believe it or not, there are actually cookbooks that have you soaking, marinating, drying and doing all kinds of time consuming things to tofu in order to make it something it is not. Why mess with it?

I'll admit that in my first introduction to whole foods, just the mention of the word "tofu" would send my eyes rolling skyward in their sockets. A little older and perhaps wiser, I hope to share some words of tofu wisdom that might help you get over your own tofu tentativeness and give it a spin yourself. Here are some tofu tactics to keep in mind:

1 Never serve tofu chunks to anyone but a small toddler.

2 If it's blended in a smoothie, that's fine. If it's floating in a smoothie, that's gross.

3 Tofu and main course should never be said in the same sentence.

4 Tasty tofu is an oxymoron.

5 Don't try and fake people out that it's meat. No one will fall for it, either will the tofu.

Everything has a purpose in life—tofu's purpose is to be healthful and good for you, not to give you gastronomic delight. Remember that next time you're seduced by a gourmet tofu recipe. Keep it simple and grab your blender. It makes a great smoothie.

Sticky Chicken

I have seen about a million recipes similar to this everywhere and they all have the same name. The reason is nothing sounds decent: sticky chicky, sticken chicken, sticket chicket....see what I mean?

Serves 4

½ cup rice wine vinegar
½ cup tamari soy sauce
¼ cup sucanat
2 cloves garlic
1 tablespoon ginger, fresh
4 chicken breasts without skin

You need to marinate these babies overnight, so while you are cleaning up the dinner dishes, get this one started for tomorrow.

In a large bag, add all ingredients except chicken. Mush the bag around to make sure the sucanat is dissolved. Add chicken and throw in the fridge. If you remember during the day, periodically shift things around so the marinade goes all over the place. But don't undo the bag to do it.

At dinner time, pull chicken from the bag and put in a large skillet, with the marinade. Bring marinade to a boil and then reduce heat to low. Cover the pan and cook about 15 minutes, turning once.

When the chicken is done, put on a plate and stick in a warm oven. There is still work to be done here!

Now turn up the heat and cook the sauce till it's almost gone. This is where the sticky part comes in. You will need to keep stirring it or it will burn easily. As a matter of fact, turn it back down to low so it doesn't burn. The entire thing should take about 10 minutes. This is called a reduction, by the way. And the sucanat sort of caramelizes it so it's a caramelized reduction already.

Now remove your warm chicken from the oven and return it to the skillet and slop them around in there to pick up that tasty sauce.

PER SERVING: 343 CALORIES (KCAL); 3G TOTAL FAT; (7% CALORIES FROM FAT); 58G PROTEIN; 19G CARBOHYDRATE; 137MG CHOLESTEROL; 2165MG SODIUM

"Our family rates foods by how often they would be willing to eat it. Sticky Chicken rated a twice a month—which is very good. I will make this again for a 'company dinner' when I want to impress someone."—Robyn St. Claire

The Magic of Marinade

This all-purpose marinade can be used for just about anything. But stick with meat and poultry, okay? Even marinades have their limitations. Makes 2 cups.

¼ cup olive oil
¾ cup tamari soy sauce
1 lemon, juiced
4 cloves garlic
3 teaspoons honey

Mix all ingredients together and use on whatever you are marinating. It's just that simple! Use a big, ol' bag to keep the mess to a minimum.

For chicken or meat, you'll want to marinate it for a few hours, even overnight in your fridge, although it depends on the cut, if there's a bone and all that. If you are cooking it indoors, try baking the chicken in a preheated 375 degree oven till it's done. And that will depend, of course, on what you have chosen to marinate and cook.

Grilling is the best method when you're working with marinades. When the coals are white-ish and red at the same time, flop your chicken (or meat) on the grill and watch it like a hawk. If you're going to go through all this trouble to marinate your dinner, you might as well eat it without it becoming a charcoal briquette.

MARINADE GUIDELINES:

• Use a Ziploc bag (as already noted)

• Make sure your meat is getting exposed to the marinade. If necessary divide up the marinade and meat into two bags.

• About 1 cup of marinade will be enough for 2-3 pounds of cut up chicken.

• Never reuse marinade. Once it's been used by the meat or chicken, it's a bacterial nightmare.

• Remember not to stick the meat or chicken back in the marinade after cooking or it will get cooties.

Variations on a Theme—To make your marinade more twangy and with bigger Asian overtones (gosh—that sounds so "food magazine," doesn't it?) Substitute sesame oil for the olive oil and rice wine vinegar for the lemon juice.

"Everyone should have a good marinade recipe like this one! This was so easy to prepare in the morning while cleaning up breakfast, then easy to pop the chicken breasts in the oven a little before supper. Grilling would be great on a hot day to keep the kitchen cool." —Michele Knoshaug

Un-Fried Chicken, My Way

Oprah would love this recipe. Oprah, if you're reading this,
I'll come on your show and cook any day of the week.

Serves 6

6 chicken breasts, skinless, boneless
1 cup skim milk
1 cup ice cubes
½ cup plain nonfat yogurt
3 egg whites
1 cup whole wheat pastry flour
2 tablespoons Paul Prudhomme's Pasta and
**   Pizza seasoning**
1 teaspoon garlic powder
1 dash sea salt

Preheat oven to 400 degrees. Coat baking sheet with oil, but go easy, not like you're trying to grease an engine.

Put the chicken in a bowl with milk and ice and let those babies soak. In another bowl, mix yogurt and egg whites well. In a bag, add flour and seasonings, shake well to mix.

To make chicken, take one piece at a time out of the milk and dip in yogurt mix, then dredge the chicken thoroughly in the seasoning mixture. Place on your greased pan. Be careful not to shake the bag to vigorously or you'll lose your yogurt! When all your pieces are breaded, pop the pan in the oven for 10-12 minutes then turn them over and cook another 10-12 minutes—depending on the thickness of the breasts. You want them done, but not so done that you could use them as roofing material either, so watch 'em (unless you need new shingles)!

PER SERVING: 313 CALORIES (KCAL); 6G TOTAL FAT; (18% CALORIES FROM FAT); 57G PROTEIN; 4G CARBOHYDRATE; 145MG CHOLESTEROL; 228MG SODIUM

"This chicken has a nice zip. My family really enjoyed it."—Christina Fredricks

Kneadless Pizza Dough

Needless to say (pun intended) you'll need a food processor for this one. In fifteen quick minutes, you'll have dough ready to go—you don't even have to let it rise!

Makes 2 crusts

1 cup warm water
2 teaspoons honey
2 teaspoons yeast
2 ½ cups whole wheat flour
2 tablespoons olive oil
1 teaspoon salt

In a measuring cup, add yeast, warm water and 1 teaspoon of the honey. Mix well and let sit for 5 minutes.

In the meantime, in a food processor bowl, add flour, oil, salt and remaining honey. Pulse to blend. Now keep the food processor running, and slowly add the yeasty water through the feed tube. Let the machine run for about a minute (this is the fake kneading part). Dough should be smooth when it's done, if not, add more flour or more water depending. Now let that dough rest about 5 minutes. You'd need a good 5 minute rest too, if you were violently spinning around a food processor for a minute.

Divide the dough in half and roll out and use according to your recipe.

PER SERVING: 110 CALORIES (KCAL); 3G TOTAL FAT; (21% CALORIES FROM FAT); 4G PROTEIN; 19G CARBOHYDRATE; 0MG CHOLESTEROL; 180MG SODIUM

"This is the simplest and tastiest pizza dough recipe I've found." —Brook Stowers

Roasted Garlic

Roast a few bulbs and keep on hand. This will jazz up even the most boring food!

**1 head garlic, slice off top to expose garlic.
    Remove any excess, papery peel.**
1 teaspoon olive oil

Slice off the tip top of the garlic head to expose garlic. Don't slice too much off!

Sit the garlic on it's root end in a casserole dish. Drizzle olive oil on the top. Cover with a lid.

Bake about an hour at 375 degrees. The heavenly scent of roasted garlic will waft all over the house. Let cool.

When you want to use it, pick it up and squeeze the soft, buttery contents out into whatever you're making—sauce, garlic bread, mashed potatoes, whatever.

PER SERVING: 44 CALORIES (KCAL); 5G TOTAL FAT; (89% CALORIES FROM FAT); TRACE PROTEIN; 1G CARBOHYDRATE; 0MG CHOLESTEROL; 1MG SODIUM

Roasted Garlic Pizza Sauce

Great sauce, easy to make, too.
Serves 12

1 bulb roasted garlic, squeeze roasted
    garlic to taste (*page 145*)
1 tablespoon olive oil
1 can plum tomatoes, 28 oz.
1 teaspoon honey
salt and pepper to taste

In a saucepan, crush tomatoes with a potato masher, add remaining ingredients and bring to a low boil. Let simmer on low for about 20 minutes.

PER SERVING: 154 CALORIES (KCAL); 2G TOTAL FAT; (10% CALORIES FROM FAT); 1G PROTEIN; 9G CARBOHYDRATE; 0MG CHOLESTEROL; 6MG SODIUM

"This sauce has terrific flavor and texture."—Christina Fredricks

"This is a terrific sauce. I'll definately make this a regular in my recipe repatoire."—Sara Pattow

Stromboli Baby

Whoever came up with the stromboli idea was a genius! This recipe must become a part of your repertoire. Not only are they a snap to make, they taste great, too. Your kids will think you've opened a pizzeria at home!
Makes about 12 strombolis

1 recipe pizza dough (pg. 143)
1 recipe pizza sauce (pg. 143)
1 pound mozzarella cheese, part skim
milk, grated
1 bunch anything else that turns your key

Preheat oven to 450 degrees. Take your dough and divide into about 10 equal parts. On a floured surface, roll out each piece of dough, blop some pizza sauce on the little dough round, whatever else you like and some cheese. Amounts are up to you, but remember, you need to be able to fold this thing in half without everything squirting out everywhere.

Fold in half, and pinch the edges closed to seal the toppings in. Bake on an ungreased cookie sheet for ten minutes or until nicely browned.

You could get the kids to help you do this—I don't know of one kid that doesn't like doing dough. But make up several batches of Kneadless Dough and keep the stromboli machine (that would be the kids) a-running! This would be a fun project and great way to fill up your freezer with good-for-you snacks and lunches—not those gross-out frozen pocket things at the grocery store.

PER RECIPE: 223 CALORIES (KCAL); 7G TOTAL FAT; (38% CALORIES FROM FAT); 12G PROTEIN; 32G CARBOHYDRATE; 2MG CHOLESTEROL; 321MG SODIUM

"Today I made the Stromboli with the help of my children. We've had a wonderful afternoon, preparing this together. It was simple, wholesome and tasty." —Kimberly Halbert

Vickilynn's Tried and True Pizza Dough

Vickilynn can cook, but in my eyes, she's the Queen of Pizza. Try this recipe and you'll see why!

Serves 16

1 ½ cups warm water
1 teaspoon honey
1 ½ teaspoons olive oil
½ teaspoon sea salt
2 cups whole wheat flour, Kamut flour can be used
2 teaspoons yeast, SAF is the best
2 tablespoons gluten, wheat additional flour for rolling out.

Mix the first 6 ingredients well. If using a mixer like a Kitchen Aid or a Bosch, add enough additional flour until the dough forms a ball and pulls away from the side of the bowl. Knead in the machine about 6-8 minutes.

If your are making this by hand, add more flour, one cup at a time mixing well after each addition until dough clings together and you can turn out on a floured surface. Knead until dough is smooth and springy about 10 -12 minutes. If you have a child with relatively clean hands or a child who can get them that way, this would be a good job for him or her. (Hint: put the timer on for this.)

Divide dough in half. If your stone does not need to be preheated, roll your dough out on the stone 1 inch wider than the stone. Turn the extra inch over the center to form a crust. Prebake it in a 500 degree oven for about 8 minutes from a cold oven and 450 for 5 minutes if oven is preheated. Do the same thing with the second crust. Then top the cooled crusts with sauce, toppings and cheese and bake at 450 for about 10-12 minutes or until the crust is brown and the toppings are cooked.

Variations: we like adding minced garlic and grated parmesan cheese as the dough is mixing. Try adding dried herbs such as basil or oregano as well.

If you prefer a thicker, breadier crust, let the dough rise on the stone after shaping until puffy then prebake and finish as directed.

No stone? Fear not. Use a cookie sheet and prebake about 5 minutes. Remove from the sheet and let cool two minutes, then put the crust right on the rack of the oven. If crust doesn't seem like it can hold up, prebake a little longer and try again. OR forget about it and make stromboli....

Freezing instructions: lightly oil the dough ball and place it in a freezer bag. Or partially bake and *then* freeze them.

PER SERVING: 65 CALORIES (KCAL); 1G TOTAL FAT; (11% CALORIES FROM FAT); 4G PROTEIN; 12G CARBOHYDRATE; 0MG CHOLESTEROL; 63MG SODIUM

COOKING NOTES: Steam some greens (see glossary if you are unsure what greens are) and then sauté the cooked greens with onion, garlic and olive oil. Try using that for fun on your pizza with the sauce and cheese and all the rest. It's a little different and really, so delicious. No one will ever suspect you tried to slip them some phytochemicals.

Just for grins, I kitchen-tested *my* tried and true pizza crust recipe. I hadn't made it for awhile since we make big batches more often, and I didn't want you having a "bomb" in your otherwise fabulous book, *and* I do have a reputation to consider!! The crust recipe worked great! I did use the olive oil and the gluten that were optional and did let it rise shortly in the bowl and on my 15 inch stone. It was thin which we like, but would be thicker on a smaller stone or pan. Whew, I am relieved it worked and my Pizza Maven rep is intact! <wiping sweat from brow>. I also whipped up a Broccoli Parmesan Pizza for the testing and thought you'd like it. Here it is, unveiled for the first time.

Broccoli Parmesan Pizzas

Vickilynn Haycraft

Topping:
2 10-ounce boxes of broccoli (not chopped). or 2 bunches fresh, cook until crisp-tender, then drain.
3 tablespoons butter
8 cloves garlic, minced (more or less to taste)
½ cup grated Parmesan cheese (or more to taste)
salt and pepper to taste
*optional; red pepper flakes, pasta seasoning etc

Mix well and spread on pre-baked crusts. Top completely with mozzarella or herbed Jack cheese. Bake in a preheated 475 degree oven for 10 minute or until cheese is bubbly.

"This is a healthy way to eat that pizza we were used to having delivered every Friday night. Quick and simple crust yet very delicious." —Lynn and Bob Saphner

Dips, Snacks & Tricks

Got a picky eater? You've come to the right place. This section is filled with dips for your sticks and tricks for lunches, snacks and other eating occasions. Nothing here is overly time consuming or takes a gourmet cook's skill. You might even employ a child or two to help. Check out Presto Pretzels and see what I mean.

Avocado Dip

Remember how to tame a picky eater? Give him a dip and a stick. Here's the dip part anyway.

Serves 20 as an appetizer

2 avocadoes, smushed
1 clove garlic, pressed
1 teaspoon soy sauce
1 cup plain low-fat yogurt
2 tablespoons dill

1 dash cayenne

Mix it all together and serve with veggies for dipping.

PER SERVING: 41 CALORIES (KCAL); 3G TOTAL FAT; (5% CALORIES FROM FAT); 1G PROTEIN; 3G CARBOHYDRATE; 1MG CHOLESTEROL; 11MG SODIUM

"A lovely, pale green dip, flecked with the darker green of the dill. Easily mixed in the food processor, it is delicious with veggies, crackers, or tortilla chips."—Lee Ann Roberts

Better Butter

This is so easy, you could make it with your eyes shut. But don't do that, you might make a mess.

Makes about 1 cup—ten tablespoons thereabouts

1 stick unsalted butter
½ cup safflower oil (or other mild tasting, cold pressed oil)

Let butter sit out to soften.

Mix together butter and oil well and store in the refrigerator in a covered container. Keeps a good while.

PER SERVING: 81 CALORIES (KCAL); 9G TOTAL FAT; (14% CALORIES FROM FAT); 1G PROTEIN; TRACE CARBOHYDRATE; 25MG CHOLESTEROL; 1MG SODIUM

"It takes a few bites to really appreciate the flavor of this butter. My first thought is to use a little less oil, because I enjoy the taste of butter, but I see the value in using less butter. This butter spreads on cornbread with ease and I really like that!"—
Marilyn May

Black Bean Dip

I was inspired to create this after eating more jars than I can calculate of Guiltless Gourmet's fabulous black bean dip. Mine is slightly different, but it is still delicious.
Serves 12 as an appetizer

1 black beans, canned, drained
1 can green chili peppers, drained
¼ cup salsa, use what you have
2 teaspoons cumin
1 teaspoon garlic, pressed
1 squeeze lime or lemon

Dump it all into a food processor and whir like mad. When it's done, blop it into a bowl and serve with any type of chip that turns your key. But preferably with a healthy one you made from these recipes.

PER SERVING: 14 CALORIES (KCAL); TRACE TOTAL FAT; (11% CALORIES FROM FAT); 1G PROTEIN; 2G CARBOHYDRATE; 0MG CHOLESTEROL; 58MG SODIUM

"We tried this last night and absolutely loved it. I was afraid they would be too hot but they were just flavorful. We used them as a dip with homemade tortilla chips and my kids rolled it up on tortillas today for lunch. They added more salsa to the tortillas and some sour cream and they were great.
Everyone has asked to have this again!" —The Beaver Family

Dip Chips

Make sure you only use the non-stick sprays from the health food store. The others are full of propellant. Propellant is fine if you have something you want to propel. In this case, I think you would prefer to eat these chips than fly them.

Serves 12

12 corn tortillas, pita bread or flour tortillas
non-stick spray (only health food stores have ones without the propellant)

Preheat oven to 425 degrees. Spray a cookie sheet generously with non-stick spray.

Stack the tortillas and cut them into 6 even pieces, sort of like a pizza. Place on the cookie sheet and lightly spray the tortillas. Bake for 8 minutes or so checking to make sure they don't get too brown.

Let cool and serve with hummus or black bean dip. Put a generous portion of veggies out with the chips, too.

PER SERVING: 56 CALORIES (KCAL); 1G TOTAL FAT; (9.6% CALORIES FROM FAT); 1G PROTEIN; 12G CARBOHYDRATE; 0MG CHOLESTEROL; 40MG SODIUM

"We all loved these!! The kids thought it was great we could have chips any time. Very easy to make!" —Tracey Kirch

Chinese Broccoli Slaw

I made this up in a panic for a potluck. Now I make it on purpose! This is a wonderful side dish that will take you all of five minutes to make.

Serves 6 or more

12 ounces broccoli slaw, prepackaged in the produce department

¼ cup cilantro, chopped fine (more if you love cilantro)

½ cup mayonnaise

2 tablespoons rice wine vinegar

1 tablespoon sesame oil

¼ cup honey-roasted peanuts

In a salad bowl, toss slaw and cilantro.

In a mixing bowl, whisk together remaining ingredients, except honey roasted peanuts.

Pour dressing over the top of slaw and toss well. Refrigerate an hour before serving so flavors can meld. Just before serving, sprinkle peanuts on top.

PER SERVING: 135 CALORIES (KCAL); 11G TOTAL FAT; (71% CALORIES FROM FAT), 2G PROTEIN; 8G CARBOHYDRATE; 0MG CHOLESTEROL; 86MG SODIUM

"This is another new favorite in our home! The sauce would be great on the typical broccoli floret salad, also."
—Marilyn May

Great Green Greens

Welcome to my world. If you live in the South, you know what greens are, if not try this out!
Servings: Depends upon how big the bunch is.

1 bunch collard greens, deribbed, chopped
turnip greens
creasy greens
kale

Wash well, derib the big ones like collards, then steam till tender. It may take awhile on the collards, the others watch. Stick a fork in to test for tenderness. Serve with rice wine vinegar. Completely delicious and highly nutritious. Definitely a high nutrient food.

PER LEAF: 11 CALORIES (KCAL); TRACE TOTAL FAT; (10% CALORIES FROM FAT); 1G PROTEIN; 2G CARBOHYDRATE; 0MG CHOLESTEROL; 7MG SODIUM

"You're right, they're Great Green Greens and I'm planting some collard greens in my garden this weekend to enjoy through the winter."—Dana O'Sullivan

Hot Spinach Dip

Everyone has had this at a party sometime in their lives, served in a big, hollowed out bread loaf.
This version is healthier and just as good!
Serves 12

1 package frozen chopped spinach, drained
1 package low-fat cream cheese
2 green onions, chopped
½ cup cheddar cheese, low-fat, shredded
1 teaspoon garlic powder
½ teaspoon Worcestershire sauce
salt and pepper

You can do this the easy way and throw everything in a crock pot and forget about it. *Or* you can do it the hard way, requiring constant stirring over a hot stove. That's all there is to that. Mix it up in a pot and stir, or mix it up in a crockpot and forget it. Crockpot should cook for 1 to 2 hours on high, stirring occasionally.

You could put this in a pinched out bread loaf or you could serve it more civilly in a bowl with some healthy chips and veggies.

One other note—why not do a double batch and freeze it? Make those indentured servants work for you!

PER SERVING: 24 CALORIES (KCAL); 1G TOTAL FAT; (29% CALORIES FROM FAT); 3G PROTEIN; 2G CARBOHYDRATE; 2MG CHOLESTEROL; 76MG SO-DIUM

"This recipe was easy and tasty."—Ginger Solomon

Hummus

Hummus is one of those things you just gotta trust me on and make.
It's delicious, especially made up like this!
Serves 6

1 can garbanzo beans, drained
2 cloves garlic
2 tablespoons lemon juice, use less lemon juice as your taste dictates
2 tablespoons tahini

Whirl it all together in a food processor, salt to taste. That's all there is to it. Just make sure you process it well. This is one of those recipes you don't want big hunks in.

COOKING NOTES: Serve as a dip with pita triangle, tortillas or the Dip Chips (page 154).

PER SERVING: 77 CALORIES (KCAL); 2G TOTAL FAT; (26% CALORIES FROM FAT); 4G PROTEIN; 11G CARBOHYDRATE; 0MG CHOLESTEROL; 7MG SODIUM

"I liked this and one of my sons loved it and requested I make it again!"—Tracey Kirch

Spinach Artichoke Dip

Another re-do on an old stand-by.

Serves 12

1 package low-fat cream cheese

¼ cup milk, 1% low-fat

½ can artichoke hearts, drained and chopped

1 package frozen chopped spinach, drained

½ cup salsa

¼ cup Romano cheese, grated

¼ cup low-fat jack cheese, grated

½ teaspoon garlic powder

In a food processor, add all ingredients and chop, chop, chop till smooth.

Heat and serve with the usual fixin's: veggies, healthy chips, cut-up bread...

COOKING NOTES: You could double this and serve at a party, give it to the kids for a fun chip-and-dip lunch. It's quick and substantial. Make sure it's smooth, no chunks allowed—chunks will probably freak out the kids.

PER SERVING: 31 CALORIES (KCAL); 1G TOTAL FAT; (32% CALORIES FROM FAT); 3G PROTEIN; 3G CARBOHYDRATE; 4MG CHOLESTEROL; 125MG SODIUM

The Ultimate Tortilla Roll-Up

You can find roll ups everywhere, even at fast food places. Here's a healthy, good-for-you spin on Roll-ups.

Serves 1

1 flour tortilla, health food stores have a sprouted wheat tortilla that is delicious

½ ounce low-fat cream cheese, you can use less

1 ounce chicken breast without skin, tuna or whatever you have on hand

2 slices tomato, chopped

1 romaine lettuce leaf, shredded

1 green onion, minced fine (optional)

1 teaspoon vinaigrette

Lay tortilla flat and spread cream cheese all over. In a small bowl, toss lettuce, tomato and optional green onion with vinaigrette. Set aside.

Lay chicken out evenly over cream cheese. Spread lettuce mixture evenly on top of the chicken.

Roll up like you would a sleeping bag and secure with a toothpick or just place on a plate, seam side down. If this is for a bag lunch, wrap securely with plastic wrap.

PER SERVING: 373 CALORIES (KCAL); 11G TOTAL FAT; (17% CALORIES FROM FAT); 16G PROTEIN; 54G CARBOHYDRATE; 21MG CHOLESTEROL; 483MG SODIUM

"This was so good!!!! My husband loved it and he didn't even catch on to the fact there was cream cheese in it! I am so surprise he looked at it like that looks weird on that tortilla and just ate it and said I love that stuff on it!"—Lori Sparks

"Light, yet filling. These versatile roll-ups make for a wonderful lunch treat. The Ultimate Tortilla Roll-Up is a very versatile lunch idea. We chose to use shredded crab instead of chicken or tuna. These are quick to prepare and perfect for lunch guests."—Susie Wietelman

Presto Pretzels

Kids are quite willing to make these for you. The mess however, is negotiable—at least in their eyes.

Serves 12

1 envelope yeast
½ cup water, warm
1 teaspoon honey
1 teaspoon sea salt
1 1/3 cups kamut flour, you could substitute whole wheat, if you would prefer
1 tablespoon gluten

Preheat oven to 400 degrees. Lightly grease cookie sheet.

In a medium-sized bowl, dissolve yeast in warm water. Add honey and salt and mix till blended.

Add flour and gluten and knead the dough till blended and doughy-like. The gluten develops better when it is kneaded well.

Roll out long pieces of dough and let the kids go nuts making whatever design they like.

Bake for 10 minutes. Loosen from the cookie sheet and let cool 5 minutes, then transfer to a wire rack to finish cooling.

PER SERVING: 88 CALORIES (KCAL); TRACE TOTAL FAT; (4% CALORIES FROM FAT); 4G PROTEIN; 20G CARBOHYDRATE; 0MG CHOLESTEROL; 158MG SODIUM

"This is a great recipe to make with kids. It is simple to mix up (my eight-year-old could handle it on his own). The shaping of the pretzels is fun for everyone, children or adults. Best of all, the results are delicious!"
—Robin Schneider

"This recipe was easy and fun for the kids. I used the whole wheat flour and it had a nice soft texture."
—Susie Wietelman

Puffy Grain Chewy Bars

This is one of those recipes that my kids beg for—it's that good. Great snack to go.
Makes 12 4x4 bars

1 cup each: Puffed kamut, brown rice, millet (you'll find these at a health food store)
½ cup peanut butter, or almond butter
½ cup honey
1 teaspoon molasses, blackstrap

Dump the cereal in a big bowl. Heat the honey, peanut butter and molasses together. Pour into cereal mixture, working quickly to get it mixed. Press firmly into a 13 X 9 inch pan. Let sit for as long as you can wait (the longer the harder) and then dig in.

COOKING NOTES: Variations of a theme: Try using brown rice crispies in place of the puffed rice, and toasting the millet and kamut on a cookie sheet (425 degree oven till toasted) for a crispy texture instead.

For more variety, use this recipe as a base and add raisins, chopped dates or chopped nuts. We tried throwing some chocolate chips in there, but they got kinda melty. Not that anyone was complaining....just thought you might like to know in case you choose to do such a thing.

PER PAN: 108 CALORIES (KCAL); 5G TOTAL FAT; (8% CALORIES FROM FAT); 3G PROTEIN; 14G CARBOHYDRATE; 0MG CHOLESTEROL; 51MG SODIUM

"Easy, chewy, sweet—a great mid-afternoon snack."—Sue LeMay

Retro Granola Bars

This recipe has definitely been reworked to be a little healthier than the 70's oily version. If you want the 70's, go for a rerun of "Charlie's Angels" or plug in a lava lamp.

Makes 24 2x2 bars

1 cup oats

¼ cup oat bran

1 cup puffed rice cereal, I use puffed brown rice cereal or brown rice crispies—either one works fine

½ cup granola, use a no-fat or low-fat granola

1 ½ cups raisins

1 ½ cups dried fruit, use whatever you have on hand. Chop up the dried fruit.

¾ cup protein powder, you can also use dried milk

¾ cup honey

½ cup almond butter, can use peanut butter instead

2 teaspoons vanilla extract

½ cup almonds, use raw and chop well

In a large bowl, put raisins, oats, puffed rice cereal, granola, dried fruit, oat bran and protein powder and toss them together.

In a medium pan, heat the honey and almond butter together till almost boiling. Add vanilla extract.

Add warm mixture to dry ingredients and mix well.

Working quickly, press the mixture into a greased 9 x 13 inch pan. Chill. Then cut into bars

PER SERVING: 160 CALORIES (KCAL); 5G TOTAL FAT; (27% CALORIES FROM FAT); 7G PROTEIN; 24G CARBOHYDRATE; 14MG CHOLESTEROL; 36MG SODIUM

"These are moist and chewy, with a nice combination of dried fruits and crispy grains for a sweet and crunchy snack. We all love them, even my two picky boys!" —Nita Crabb

Teriyaki Salmon

This is fast food like no other. You'll love it!
Serves 4

4 salmon fillets
4 tablespoons teriyaki sauce, use low sodium

Preheat broiler in oven.

Wash fillets and blot with paper towel. On a cookie sheet, evenly distribute filets.

Put one tablespoon of the sauce evenly on each salmon filet. You can allow the fish to marinate a bit, but it's not necessary, although I prefer to allow the sauce to soak in at least an hour before cooking.

Broil fish but watch like a hawk. You don't want it to burn. If it's too close, move it. Entire cooking should be around 6 minutes, depending on how thick your salmon is.

PER SERVING: 212 CALORIES (KCAL); 6G TOTAL FAT; (25% CALORIES FROM FAT); 35G PROTEIN; 3G CARBOHYDRATE; 88MG CHOLESTEROL; 804MG SODIUM

Just Desserts

There are certain moments in life when dinner should be capped off with something sweet. That doesn't mean everyday or even once a week. Remember I mentioned earlier that we need to take seriously the need to retrain our voracious sweet tooths (teeth?). But to say good bye to dessert forever? May it never be! A delightful apple crisp to celebrate those first days of fall is reason enough to bake this wonderful dessert and everyone needs to try the Maple Flan at least once. Honest —enjoy them all. Just not too often.

Amber's Friend Nina's Cookies

Quite a cookie...great for lunch boxes and they store well. Makes 36 Cookies

2 bananas, ripe

2 eggs

½ cup peanut butter

½ cup raisins

1 cup nuts and seeds, try: almonds, sunflower seeds, walnuts, pumpkin seeds—all raw

½ cup dry milk, or skip if dairy is an issue

1 teaspoon baking powder

½ cup each oat flour, kamut, whole wheat

½ teaspoon baking soda

½ cup oatmeal

½ cup wheat germ

½ cup pumpkin puree

½ cup chocolate chips, Sunspire brand, grain sweetened.

1 tablespoon blackstrap molasses

In a bowl, smash two bananas, add eggs, peanut butter, pumpkin, honey and molasses. Mix well. Then add powdered milk and other dry ingredients and mix well. If it seems too stiff, add a little water. You want the consistency of regular, ol' drop cookies, like peanut butter cookies. Add the chocolate chips, raisins and nuts. Again, a little water if it's too stiff. This isn't an exact, have to be on the mark, recipe. You don't want it to be runny, but you certainly want to be able to move your wooden spoon through the mixture without putting your shoulder out of socket.

Drop on to an ungreased cookie sheet and bake till nice and brown, but not too brown.

At this point, you're probably thinking, "Okay, I can do that, but what temp?" Glad you asked. Make that a 350 degree preheated oven.

PER COOKIE: 73 CALORIES (KCAL); 4G TOTAL FAT; (42% CALORIES FROM FAT); 3G PROTEIN; 9G CARBOHYDRATE; 12MG CHOLESTEROL; 59MG SODIUM

Amber says, "These are wonderful! My kids eat these like they are going to run away or something, and they are getting a ton of fiber and protein."

"These cookies are packed full of healthy ingredients. This is one cookie I actually encourage my daughter to eat."—Deborah Hockman

Substitutions, Hints & Stuff

Every one of the recipes in this book have all been tested, tasted and passed by the Healthy-Foods taste testers (and their families) and by my own family. A lot of the recipes had to be tested, rewritten and tested again, simply because I am the type of cook that measures nothing—not even muffins. I have an idea of proportions, what it should look like then I just dump stuff into a bowl and more often than not, I'm quite pleased with the results.

I recognize though, that not everyone is comfortable with such "methodology" and have provided things like measurements, sizes of pans and oven temperatures. In any case, the whole point of what I'm getting at is, don't be caught up in the running-off-to-the-store-thing if you don't have an ingredient. There are certain things that are essential, obviously, but there are certain things that aren't.

Here's a quick guide for doing things YOUR way, whether or not the recipe tells you can or cannot. Recipes are a lot more flexible than we give them credit for, so remember that if you run out of something mid-recipe.

Substitutions

Buttermilk—use milk and add a couple of teaspoon-fuls of vinegar or lemon. I use buttermilk a lot because it gives a dish a lot of complexity and richness without all the fat. Obviously, substitute something non-dairy if milk allergies are an issue.

Milk—soy milks and rice milks can easily be used instead of dairy milk. If you'll notice, I don't mention soy cheese or soy yogurt in the book. That's because they taste nasty. Maybe there is one out there that is decent, but thus far my quest for non-dairy cheeses and yogurts has reaped nothing but a gross aftertaste.

Peanut butter or almond butter—either or works fine—same proportions. For a great sandwich, try almond butter, honey and sliced banana on whole wheat bread...yum.

Chicken broth—can be exchanged for vegetable broth or try the roasted vegetable stock recipe in this book.

Butter—use a little oil instead or skip it entirely. Spectrum Naturals has a non-trans fatty acid margarine if you prefer a no-dairy spread. I cannot tell you what it tastes like though.

Sucanat—most of my dessert recipes call for sucanat. (see glossary if you don't know what it is) For most recipes, you could probably get away with honey, but about half as much since it's much sweeter.

Safflower oil—oils are best when they are not cooked. However, adding a little bit of oil to a baked good makes all the difference. Although safflower is the best oil (because of the almost non-flavor) for baking with, olive oil is healthier.

Beans—you can get them dried or canned. Sometimes I call for canned in a recipe, sometimes I call for dried that you make up yourself. The point is using them how you have them. If you have a ton cooked and in the freezer, please don't run out and buy a can of beans! And don't cook any up if you happen to have a case of Y2K beans in your linen closet. For cooked, just measure out about 1¼ cups per "can" and call it a day.

Mayonnaise—boy, the choices available today—nonfat, low-fat, mayonnaise, regular...yikes. Makes a gal dizzy. My suggestion is you use what you like. The full fat stuff isn't exactly great for you, the nonfat stuff is made from weird stuff...a low-fat, premium brand with ingredients you can pronounce is probably the best tactic, although there are other decent mayos from the health food store available.

Apple Cake

I don't like a cake with raisins and nuts in it, either do my kids. However, there is an active raisin and nut loving contingent in the population so I have made a note in the directions on how you can add them.

Serves 12

1 egg
2 egg whites
¼ cup safflower oil
2 teaspoons vanilla extract
1 cup maple syrup
1 ½ cups whole wheat pastry flour
¾ cup whole wheat flour
2 teaspoons cinnamon
2 teaspoons baking soda
3 cups apple, chopped
½ cup buttermilk, or soy milk with a
   teaspoon of vinegar
2 tablespoons organic sucanat

Preheat oven to 325 degrees. Prepare a 9 inch square pan by greasing.

Chop apples and toss with the sucanat. Set aside

Beat together eggs, maple syrup, vegetable oil and vanilla.

In a large bowl, toss together all dry ingredients. Make a well in the center and mix wet stuff in well.

Add the chopped apples to the batter and optional nuts and raisins. (½ cup each)

Bake for about 1 hour, maybe a little more, until a toothpick inserted in the middle comes out clean.

Let cool in the pan for at least 10 minutes, then remove it carefully and finish cooling on a rack. For a special occasion, top with cream cheese frosting (*see page 175*).

PER SERVING: 175 CALORIES (KCAL); 5G TOTAL FAT; (26% CALORIES FROM FAT); 2G PROTEIN; 31G CARBOHYDRATE; 16MG CHOLESTEROL; 237MG SODIUM

"For breakfast we had apple cake and we loved it!" —Lori Sparks

Juicy Jello

Besides the added flavor and taste, using a juice combo instead of plain apple juice
will make this treat look a lot better!
Servings: It all depends on how you slice it.

1 tablespoon unflavored gelatin
¼ cup water
1 ½ cups fruit juice combination, apple
   boysenberry juice or some kind of
   combo is good.
¼ cup apple juice, frozen concentrate

Mix gelatin and water in a medium bowl: let stand to soften (about 1 minute).

Bring juice to a boil in a saucepan. Add juice to gelatin mixture and stir until completely dissolved.

Pour mixture into 8 inch square baking dish and chill till firm. Cut into cubes and serve.

PER RECIPE: 173 CALORIES (KCAL); TRACE TOTAL FAT; (1% CALORIES FROM FAT); 2G PROTEIN; 42G CARBOHYDRATE; 0MG CHOLESTEROL; 57MG SODIUM

"My kids and I loved this." —Lori Sparks

Awesome Apple Crisp

Close to what my mom used to make——without the white sugar.
Serves 6 generously

5 cups Granny Smith apples, chopped
½ cup sucanat——more or less depending on
the sweetness of your apples
1 ½ teaspoons cinnamon
½ cup whole wheat pastry flour
½ cup oats
¼ cup unsalted butter
1 teaspoon vanilla extract

In a large bowl, put your chopped apples, a ½ cup of sucanat and cinnamon and mix well.

In a food processor, process the pastry flour, oats, remaining sucanat, butter and vanilla pulsing just to blend. You want it lumpy and bumpy, not smooth. (Actually, if you really want to push the envelope a little here, double the recipe for the topping and go for it. It is sooo good!)

Preheat oven to 375 degrees. Put ½ cup of topping in with the apples and toss well.

Fill a 2-quart baking dish with apples and top with remaining topping. Bake for 35 minutes till browned nicely.

Serve in bowls with some vanilla yogurt on top or some cold milk.

PER SERVING: 237 CALORIES (KCAL); 9G TOTAL FAT; (31% CALORIES FROM FAT); 3G PROTEIN; 40G CARBOHYDRATE; 21MG CHOLESTEROL; 3MG SODIUM

"This looked, smelled, and tasted great! The whole family liked it. I definitely plan to make it again."
—Bonnie Musselwhite

"Two thumbs up for Awesome Apple Crisp, this recipe is guaranteed to please the bunch!" —Susie Wietelman

Baked Cinnamon Apples

The smell of these cooking is reason enough to make them.
Serves 4

4 Granny Smith apples, cored
1 teaspoon cinnamon
¼ teaspoon nutmeg
4 teaspoons organic sucanat
2 teaspoons unsalted butter

Preheat oven to 350 degrees. Take apples and set them in a Pyrex dish. Sprinkle spices and sucanat on the apple and top with ½ teaspoon of butter each. Bake for about 45 minutes. Serve warm with vanilla yogurt.

Tastes like a rich, apple-y custard without all that nasty fat—that little bit of butter makes them almost velvety in texture and rich in flavor. If you want a little bit of nasty fat, go to Awesome Apple Crisp and knock yourself out...

PER SERVING: 100 CALORIES (KCAL); 2G TOTAL FAT; (17% CALORIES FROM FAT); TRACE PROTEIN; 21G CARBOHYDRATE; 5MG CHOLESTEROL; 3MG SODIUM

"The apples smelled wonderful while they were cooking. The kids loved them and happily begged for more. It was nice to know they are good for you. Perfect holiday dish!"—Lori Sparks

Bread Pudding

There is nothing like a bowl of warm bread pudding and cuddling with a story by the fire.

Serves 8

6 slices whole grain bread
3 eggs
2/3 cup sucanat
2 teaspoons vanilla
unsalted butter
2 ½ cups milk

Preheat oven to 350 degrees. Butter the bread on both sides and place in a greased 9 X 5 loaf pan.

You should have built a little bread wall in there. Now mix up the other ingredients and pour over the top. Stick in another pan (we're doing that ban marie thing again—see Maple Flan on page 182 if you need an explanation) and pour boiling water in till it reaches half way up the pan. Very carefully, put the pan into the oven.

Bake about 45 minutes. This is definitely one of those desserts that warrants being checked on. You want tender bread pudding. NOT the texture of banana bread.

When finished baking, remove from the oven and the water bath and let rest till coolish. Serve sliced with raspberry sauce slathered on top.

COOKING NOTES: Serve with a raspberry puree. To make, dump a bag of frozen raspberries into a blender with a teeny, tiny bit of honey and about ¼ cup of water. You're sort of on your own here and you'll have to experiment a bit with flavor and thickness. Not all frozen raspberries are created equal.

PER SERVING: 226 CALORIES (KCAL); 6G TOTAL FAT; (21% CALORIES FROM FAT); 8G PROTEIN; 38G CARBOHYDRATE; 80MG CHOLESTEROL; 224MG SODIUM

"The kids and I made the bread pudding and it was great. I was concerned that it would be bland without any cinnamon or raisins. The kids thought it was good just the way it was. It was so easy to make my 11 and 12 year old boys made one the next night all by themselves. We used fresh raspberries in the sauce and didn't need any honey at all. The kids ate both the raspberry sauce, and when that ran out, used leftover chocolate pudding on top!"

—Kathy Beaver

Carrot Cake

Morbidly rich, reserve for very special occasions.
This shouldn't be standard stuff at all. (although, every once in awhile won't hurt...)
Serves 12

¼ cup safflower oil
1 cup organic sucanat
2 cups whole wheat pastry flour
1 teaspoon nutmeg
2 teaspoons cinnamon
1 teaspoon baking soda
1 teaspoon baking powder
1 teaspoon sea salt
2 each eggs
4 cups carrots, grated
1 cup pecans, chopped
1 teaspoon vanilla extract

Preheat your oven to 350 degrees. Prepare a 9 x 12 inch pan by greasing well.

In a large bowl, mix oil and sucanat together, add eggs one at a time till mixed well. Set aside.

In another bowl, mix all dry ingredients well.

Make a well in the dry ingredients and add the wet ingredients. When mixed, add carrots, vanilla extract and pecans.

Pour into prepared pan and bake for an hour. Test for doneness. If its still goopy in the middle, bake another 10 minutes.

This is one of those leave-it-in-the-pan cakes. Top with cream cheese frosting *(page 175)* if you really want to knock yourself out.

PER SERVING: 207 CALORIES (KCAL); 12G TOTAL FAT; (47% CALORIES FROM FAT); 2G PROTEIN; 26G CARBOHYDRATE; 31MG CHOLESTEROL; 327MG SODIUM

"My kids told me 'we loved the cake even with the carrots!'
I thought it was very moist which I like!" —Lori Sparks

Cream Cheese Frosting

This can be used for about anything. If you're desperate, just use a spoon and skip the cake.
Enough for one 13x9 cake

6 ounces low-fat cream cheese
1 tablespoon unsalted butter
3 tablespoons honey
1 tablespoon vanilla

In a small bowl, mix all ingredients together. Refrigerate till ready to use.

COOKING NOTES: You can use this on top of carrot cake, zucchini bread (made into a cake), cinna-buns, the whole shebang.

PER SERVING: 60 CALORIES (KCAL); 3G TOTAL FAT; (51% CALORIES FROM FAT); 2G PROTEIN; 6G CARBOHYDRATE; 11MG CHOLESTEROL; 99MG SODIUM

Crockpot Applesauce

Tastes like warm apple pie. It's heavenly made with Galas and no sweetener is required.
Serves 6

3 pounds Gala or Jonathan apples, peeled and quartered
1 cinnamon stick or 1½ teaspoons cinnamon

In a crockpot, place prepared apples and cinnamon and cook on high for about 3 hours, or until fork tender. Serve in bowls warm.

For an extra special touch, put about a half teaspoon of butter on top and sprinkle with a little bit of sucanat.

PER SERVING: 105 CALORIES (KCAL); 1G TOTAL FAT; (1% CALORIES FROM FAT); TRACE PROTEIN; 28G CARBOHYDRATE; 0MG CHOLESTEROL; 5MG SODIUM

"We used Gala apples. This recipe gets a 10 in easy preparation and great taste. It tastes somewhere between apple pie without the crust and apple cider with texture." —Carol Reynolds

Gretel's Gingerbread

Whatever happened to those crazy kids, Hansel and Gretel? Well, Hansel began a computer start up, GBHouse.com and is now independently wealthy. In the meantime, Gretel is making organic gingerbread and making a fortune selling it over the internet, in between doing the wash and carpool. This is a heavier-type gingerbread because of the kamut flour. However, it wouldn't be a big deal to lighten it up using all whole wheat pastry flour.

Serves 12

1 cup kamut flour
½ cup whole wheat pastry flour
1 tsp. baking soda
1 tsp. baking powder
2 teaspoons cinnamon
2 teaspoons ginger
1 egg white
1 egg
¼ cup safflower oil
¾ cup buttermilk
1 tablespoon blackstrap molasses
½ cup honey

Preheat oven to 350 degrees and prepare a 8 inch square pan by lightly greasing.

In a large bowl, mix well dry ingredients. Make a well in the middle.

In a medium bowl, beat eggs well and remaining ingredients. Add to dry ingredients incorporating well.

Pour into prepared pan and bake for about 25 to 30 minutes, or until a toothpick inserted in the middle comes out clean.

Cool completely before cutting. For an extra special treat, top with cream cheese frosting (see *page 175*).

PER SERVING: 164 CALORIES (KCAL); 5G TOTAL FAT; (27% CALORIES FROM FAT); 4G PROTEIN; 28G CARBOHYDRATE; 16MG CHOLESTEROL; 27MG SODIUM

"Gretel's Gingerbread is moist and slightly chewy, with a delightful ginger zest. It would be great to take to a picnic or barbecue. My family devoured the whole pan in about five minutes!" —Lee Ann Roberts

Harvest Apple Bars

These look like more of a production than they really are. This is something your kids will love, and if you can keep from snitching a bite or two, you're a better woman than I.

Serves 12

2 cups whole wheat pastry flour
1 cup oatmeal
1 teaspoon vanilla extract
¼ cup sucanat
5 apples, peeled, diced
2 teaspoons cinnamon
1 teaspoon vanilla extract
¼ cup sucanat
¼ cup whole wheat pastry flour
½ teaspoon nutmeg
1 stick unsalted butter, sliced ½" thick

Preheat oven to 350 degrees. Grease a 9x13 pan.

In a food processor, pulse the flour, oats and sucanat until mixed. Add cold butter. Pulse until blended and it looks like granola. Then pulse some more till you get a nice dough. Press the dough into the prepared pan. Bake for about 12 minutes or so till dough is set, not browned.

Make the filling with the apples, pastry flour, sucanat, vanilla and cinnamon. Toss together well and spread evenly over the cooled crust.

Bake for about 40 minutes or until the apples are done and the crust is browned, but not burnt.

Serve with a little vanilla yogurt or whipped cream.

Makes 24 bars (2 x 3")

PER SERVING: 64 CALORIES (KCAL); 4G TOTAL FAT; (56% CALORIES FROM FAT); 1G PROTEIN; 7G CARBOHYDRATE; 10MG CHOLESTEROL; 1MG SODIUM

"My family really enjoyed these!" —Marya Mesa

"Very good flavor—would taste great with a low-fat sour cream layer, or maybe crumbled over frozen yogurt. Definitely a keeper" —Marcella Burns

Mama's PMS Cake

Okay, picture this. I'm working on the book (yes, this one), I'm in my sweats, tired of looking at a computer screen and writing about healthy stuff. My mind turns to wicked chocolate thoughts——A Cake Is Born

Serving Size: 1

(Ah, I'm sort of kidding about the serving size. You see, if you choose to make this at a reasonable hour of the day, you'll have to share. If not, and you decide to make it at say, midnight, snarf it down and don't confess. Hide the evidence in the oven and don't say a word, but make sure you aren't walking around with dried batter on your chin——at that point, the gig is up.)

2 cups whole wheat pastry flour
1 cup organic sucanat
1 cup buttermilk
1 teaspoon vanilla extract
¼ cup unsalted butter, melted
¼ cup unsweetened cocoa
2 each eggs
½ cup chocolate chips, or more if needed
2 teaspoons baking soda
1 teaspoon sea salt
1 teaspoon baking powder

In a large bowl, mix all dry ingredients and make a well.

In a medium-sized bowl, beat eggs together with butter, buttermilk and vanilla.

Pour into a greased 13 x 9 pan and sprinkle as many chocolate chips as you need to all over the top. Bake in a preheated oven of 350 degrees for about 20-30 minutes or until a toothpick inserted in the middle comes out clean.

Decent people let it cool for at least 5 minutes before burying their faces in it. At least attempt the cool down period.

PER SERVING: 2160 CALORIES (KCAL); 92G TOTAL FAT; (36% CALORIES FROM FAT); 29G PROTEIN; 335G CARBOHYDRATE; 507MG CHOLESTEROL; 3252MG SODIUM

"Moist and lightly sweet—I would invent a case of PMS just so I'd have an excuse to make this cake!"
—Lee Ann Roberts

A Chocolate Confessional

No mystery here. I haven't exactly hidden my monthly penchant for chocolate from anyone. I admit to a piece here and again, especially at "certain times." As a matter of fact, there are moments in life when nothing will do but a Kit-Kat bar.

I have come to the conclusion that this overt fondness of chocolate is hereditary. My daughter has emerged in her own right, right out of the chocolate gene pool to claim her own spot in this accursed sisterhood. It seriously frightens me, but at least I'm empathetic.

If I have eaten chocolate within the last week, she'll smell it on my breath. "Aha!" she'll exclaim. "Where is it?" No one within earshot knows what "it" could possibly mean, unless of course, they are One of Us. Like pod people from the movie, "Invasion of the Body Snatchers", we know right away what "it" is.

"It," of course, refers to the Reese's Pieces in my desk drawer, next to the paper clips.

With recipes named "Death by Chocolate", is there nothing a chocoholic won't do to satisfy the passion for chocolate? Even the internet isn't safe for chocolate addicts. Case in point: www.virtualchocolate.com.

"I like chocolate. I was electrocuted because I started to lick the monitor," (quote from the website). That's one way to accomplish "death by chocolate". This website has anything you could ever dream of in the chocolate department—chocolate desserts, candy—the kind that can be easily sent to chocolate addict friends anywhere in the world-via email. Melts on the screen, not in your hands.

That's right—chocolate courtesy of the World Wide Web. At least this kind of chocolate won't leave you with www.poundstolose.com.

But look here, there are Rules of Chocolate. If you happen to live with a chocoholic, you'd best learn these quick. Your very life could depend on it:

1 To err is human—but if you mess with my chocolate, you're history.

2 Chocolate flavored chocolate is an abomination. Give us only the Real Thing.

3 If it's imported, in a gold box and cost half your paycheck, we'll follow you anywhere.

4 National Chocolate Day—could be as frequently as once a month. Be prepared.

5 Hershey Kisses, human kisses—if you're sensitive, don't ask which ones we like better.

Chocolate soothes the savage beast as chocolate addict will tell you and at long last, there is finally medical proof. Catechins, the antioxidants found in green tea that everyone's been talking about as being the latest and greatest anticancer fighting component, is found in greater abundance in chocolate! Four times greater, according to Holland's National Institute of Public Health and Environment. Leave it to the Dutch to come up with this research—the world's finest chocolate producers.

So rejoice! You now have a legitimate excuse for your monthly indulgence.

Remember that next time you're caught eating from a one pound bag of M & M's in the car. Just tell them you're trying to give your immune system a boost. If they're even remotely in touch with the latest health news, they'll understand.

Maple Flan

This is really just a baked custard, but doesn't Maple Flan sound so elegant and difficult to make?
Serves 8

4 eggs, beaten
½ cup maple syrup
2 teaspoons vanilla extract
**3 cups milk, 2% low-fat, heated, till almost
    boiling**
1 tablespoon sucanat

Preheat oven to 350 degrees. In the meantime, put the kettle on. You will need about 4 cups of hot water.

In a bowl, whisk together eggs, syrup and vanilla. Heat milk till almost boiling and slowly stir it into the egg mixture.

Fill individual custard cups and set in a 2-quart casserole dish. Sprinkle the tops with sucanat. Carefully pour hot water into the casserole dish till the water comes up about half way to the individual custard cups. This is known as a bain marie (water bath).

Carefully place your little flan friends in the oven and bake 45 to 50 minutes. The edges will be cooked but the middle might still look a little uncooked, but fear not, it will finish cooking, so take it out. You don't want it overcooked or it will become the texture of tofu and that's not a good thing.

Let cool and refrigerate. Serve chilled or if you just can't wait, eat it warm!

PER SERVING: 140 CALORIES (KCAL); 4G TOTAL FAT; (25% CALORIES FROM FAT); 6G PROTEIN; 20G CARBOHYDRATE; 100MG CHOLESTEROL; 75MG SODIUM

"A light, delicately flavored custard that received rave reviews from my children"—Christina Fredricks

Mama's Brown Rice Pudding

*This is what Mama would have made if brown rice were available—
you know she would love this homey dessert!*

Serves 6

1 cup brown rice, cooked
½ cup maple syrup
1 ¾ cups milk, 1% low-fat
1 egg
3 egg whites
½ teaspoon cinnamon
¼ teaspoon nutmeg
½ cup raisins

Cook the rice according to package directions, or 2:1 ratio—2 cups water to one cup rice.

In a medium saucepan, beat remaining ingredients together (except raisins). Add cooked rice and cook for about 10 minutes over medium to low heat. Watch your pot.

Ladle into individual serving dishes and top with a little sucanat and cinnamon, if you like.

PER SERVING: 270 CALORIES (KCAL); 2G TOTAL FAT; (8% CALORIES FROM FAT); 8G PROTEIN; 55G CARBOHYDRATE; 34MG CHOLESTEROL; 78MG SODIUM

"It is delicious....and so simple!! The kids (with the exception of my 11 year old that thinks that any rice pudding looks like worm pudding!) are in the other room polishing it off now. Even my very cautious husband liked it."—Dinah Luevano

Peanut Butter Cookies

These are totally wonderful. An adaptation of a well known recipe.
Makes 3 dozen cookies

1 cup peanut butter, the oily kind with the oil floating on top

1 cup sucanat

1 egg, beaten

1 ½ teaspoons vanilla extract

½ teaspoon sea salt

½ teaspoon baking soda

2 cups whole wheat pastry flour

1/8 cup unsalted butter

¼ cup peanuts

Cream peanut butter, sucanat and butter together. Preheat oven to 350. Lightly grease cookie sheets.

In a separate bowl, sift together salt, baking soda and flour. Stir dry ingredients into peanut butter mixture. Drop by teaspoonfuls on to cookie sheets. Lightly press dough down and press about 4 peanuts into the top of each cookie. This is totally optional, but adds a nice crunch.

Bake for 10-12 minutes. Let cool on cookie sheet about 5 minutes, then loosen with a spatula and transfer to a wire rack to finish cooling.

PER COOKIE: 56 CALORIES (KCAL); 5G TOTAL FAT; (8% CALORIES FROM FAT); 2G PROTEIN; 2G CARBOHYDRATE; 7MG CHOLESTEROL; 79MG SODIUM

Really High Fluffy Berry Pie

Good stuff. Sweet, fluffy pie. Hits the spot.
Serves 8

1 envelope unflavored gelatin
2 tablespoons honey
½ cup water
1 ½ cups frozen mixed berries, pureed in a blender
12 ounces low-fat cream cheese, at room temperature

In a saucepan, stir gelatin, honey and water together. Let sit for a couple of minutes. At that point, heat the mixture, stirring constantly until the gelatin is dissolved and the mixture starts to come to a boil.

Transfer the mixture to a mixing bowl and add cream cheese and berry puree. Mix well on high with electric beaters. Put this mixture back in the fridge to chill for a bit, but not to set, maybe an hour. Pour this mixture into a prepared variation of the whole wheat pie crust (see *page 186*) and chill pie for a few hours or till set.

PER SERVING: 117 CALORIES (KCAL); 7G TOTAL FAT; (57% CALORIES FROM FAT); 5G PROTEIN; 7G CARBOHYDRATE; 24MG CHOLESTEROL; 299MG SODIUM

"Fruity, light, refreshing—really a delicious summer treat."—Sue LeMay

Whole Wheat Pie Crust

This was the last thing I changed in my journey to healthy eating. I gotta tell you, a can of shortening sure does a number on a pie crust, like nothing else. Well, till this pie crust anyway.

Serves 16

2 ½ cups whole wheat pastry flour
3 tablespoons unsalted butter, cut into 1"
 pieces
2 tablespoons safflower oil
2 tablespoons ice water, plus 1 tablespoon
pinch sea salt
2 teaspoons sucanat, optional (see notes)

Measure flour and place in a food processor. Add the butter pieces and process, pulsing till blended and resembling coarse meal. Add oil and repeat the process.

Now begin adding the ice water, trickling it through the feed tube with the motor running. The mixture should begin forming a ball and when it gets to that point, stop. This isn't bread, it's pie crust and too much handling will toughen the poor thing right out. If it's a big sticky ball though, you'll need to add a little more flour and process a wee bit more. Key words are: wee bit. Just enough so it's not sticky.

Now transfer the dough to a big sheet of plastic wrap and top with another big sheet. Flatten it into a big disc and refrigerate for at least an hour. The disc shape makes rolling out so much easier.

When you're ready for the roll out, make sure you have a nice floured surface and don't over handled it. This is pie crust, remember?

To prebake a pie crust, preheat the oven to 425 degrees. Roll out and line a 9" pie pan, allowing about ½" to come off the sides, then pinch to make the crust. Prick the crust all over gently with a fork and bake for 12-15 minutes.

COOKING NOTES: Variations on a theme: For a scrumptious dessert crust, you can add about ½ cup almonds and a heaping teaspoon or two of sucanat in place of ¼ cup of the flour. Make sure you process it well.

PER SERVING: 34 CALORIES (KCAL); 4G TOTAL FAT; (99% CALORIES FROM FAT); TRACE PROTEIN; TRACE CARBOHYDRATE; 6MG CHOLESTEROL; TRACE SODIUM

"The crust has a nutty whole grain flavor that's versatile for any pie loving family seeking a healthier alternative to traditional crusts."—Dana O'Sullivan

Zippy Zucchini Bread

This zuccini bread defies description, but let's give it a try anyway. Luscious, languid, lovely....you get the idea.

2 Loaves

1 cup organic sucanat

2 egg whites

1 egg

½ cup applesauce, unsweetened

½ cup buttermilk

¼ cup oil

1 cup whole wheat flour

1 cup whole wheat pastry flour

1 teaspoon baking soda

2 teaspoons baking powder

1 ½ teaspoons cinnamon

1 teaspoon vanilla

1 ½ cups zucchini, shredded

½ cup pecans, chopped

Preheat oven to 350 degrees. Grease 2 loaf pans.

In a large bowl, mix all dry ingredients well, except sucanat.

Mix eggs together till foamy, add oil, buttermilk, applesauce and sucanat. Beat till incorporated. Add vanilla.

Make a well in the center of the dry ingredients and add wet ingredients. Mix well, but don't overdo it.

Pour batter into both pans and bake for 45 to 55 minutes.

Cool in pans, then carefully remove from pans and cool on a rack.

PER SERVING: 100 CALORIES (KCAL); 4G TOTAL FAT; (35% CALORIES FROM FAT); 2G PROTEIN; 15G CARBOHYDRATE; 8MG CHOLESTEROL; 106MG SODIUM

"This was one our favorite zucchini bread recipes, and we love zucchini bread! I used honey instead of sucanat and the flavor was wonderful. It was a beautiful loaf with a golden brown color. This was something I'd be happy to present to friends as gifts."—Jen Pitoniak

Resources

Here are some valuable resources I use myself and highly recommend. The list is short because it's only stuff I know, have used and would say without a shadow of a doubt—buy this, use this or sign up for this:

Cool Fruits—*Finally,* you get great, healthy snack stuff via the internet. www.coolfruits.com as mentioned in *Snack Attack* on page 97. Great tasting, fun snacks—nothing to make!

Co-op list: www.coopdirectory.org This list provides different co-op's available throughout the United States. For a little work and help in the co-op, you can usually get your health food store stuff less inexpensively.

Cheri Swanson, C.N.C available for consults on the telephone. My mentor, and all around great gal. Gotta love Cheri. She is also the one to call for supplements. (949) 640-9089.

Healthy-Foods: This is my own ezine that I send out weekly. It's free and always full of up-to-the-minute health news, some good recipes or ideas and great guest columns. To join, send an email to: Join-healthy-foods @xc.org

Kashi: Some really great cereals come from a company called Kashi. Where I live, it's hard to find the whole line, but now you can buy all of Kashi's wonderful cereals on the internet at www.kashi.com. If you have never had this incredible cereal, you're missing out. From the breakfast pilaf to my favorite, Kashi Good Friends, their cereals are just fabulous. They have their Kashi club on their site, that you can join free and get recipes and coupons...it's great. Or write to them at Kashi Company, P.O. Box 8557, La Jolla, CA 92038-8557

Frozen Assets Lite and Easy by Deborah Taylor-Hough (www.championpress.com). Debi has lightened up her timesaving message—Cook for a day and eat for a month. Great tips on how to pull this freezer cooking thing off. Debi is the Queen of Frozen Assets and her knowledge is indispensable, especially if your goal is to fill your freezer with meals. Check out her website: www.simplemom.com. From there, you can navigate to her other free resources: newsletters, tips, etc. An invaluable resource.

Naturally Healthy Living: Real Food For Real Families (Loyal Publishing) 1-888-77-LOYAL. Shonda Parker and Vickilynn Haycraft, authors. This book is co-authored by Vickilynn, one of our taste testers! Vickilynn is an excellent cook and wrote the recipe section to the *Naturally Healthy Living* book. Great resource. Shonda also produces a magazine called Naturally Healthy, for which Vickilynn writes a regular column. Vickilynn's website is: http://home-educate.com/WFD, Shonda's is www.naturallyhealthy.org

Village Organics—another internet site that will get you what your health food store might not have—and they deliver! www.villageorganics.com

Skeet and Ike's—soybean nuts in a variety of flavors with new stuff coming soon: www.skeetike.com

References

Schachter, Michael, M.D. F.A.C.A.M. "The Dangers of Fluoride and Fluoridation." *HealthWorld Online* http://www.healthy.net/asp/templates/article/ 540.html.

Carson, Rachel. *Silent Spring.* New York: Houghton Mifflin, 1994

Worthington, Virginia Sc.D. "A Fresh Look at an Old Debate." *Acres USA.* Austin, Texas: June, 1998.

Organic Gardening. Emmaus, Pennsylvania: May/June 1997

Cowley, Geoffrey. "Generation XXL." *Newsweek,* July 3, 2000, pp. 40-44

Rapp, Doris, M.D. *Is This Your Child?* New York: William Morrow & Company, 1992

Hornblow, Deborah. "Commentary: Good Table Manners Begin at Dinner with Proper Training from Parents." *Hartford Courant,* June 30, 1998

Index

PLEASE VISIT WWW.CHAMPIONPRESS.COM
TO LEARN MORE ABOUT LEANNE ELY'S OTHER BOOKS:

The Frantic Family Cookbook: mostly healthy meals in minutes
and the
Healthy Food Unit Study: a child's guide to nutrition and wellness

YOU'LL ALSO FIND MANY OTHER GREAT
COOKBOOKS AND LIFESTYLE TITLES, SUCH AS

- *Home Management 101: a guide for busy parents*
- *The Complete Crockery Cookbook: create spectacular meals in your slow cooker*
- *The Rush Hour Cook's Weekly Wonders: 19 weekly meal plans complete with shopping lists*
- *Frozen Assets Lite & Easy: how to cook for a day and eat for a month*
- *Squeezing Your Size 14 Self Into a Size 6 World: a real-woman's guide to food, fitness and self-acceptance*
- *Power Desserts: the ultimate collection of low-fat indulgences*

YOU MAY ALSO ENJOY...

www.womeninwellness.com
Stop by and join this free wellness community for women!